The Steps a Young Woman Must Take

Written by
Clara D. Anderson

Illustrated by
William Wynn

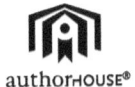

authorHOUSE®

AuthorHouse™
1663 Liberty Drive
Bloomington, IN 47403
www.authorhouse.com
Phone: 1-800-839-8640

First published by AuthorHouse 7/3/2009

ISBN: 978-1-4389-9911-1 (e)
ISBN: 978-1-4389-9909-8 (sc)
ISBN: 978-1-4389-9910-4 (hc)

Printed in the United States of America
Bloomington, Indiana

This book is printed on acid-free paper.

To

Maliyah A. McClarin, Leia K. Bozeman

Alecia K. Hill, Taiymeeka Brown,

Makia Lynn, Susanne Lynn,

Jabrielle R. Parks, Joi' Tate, Bonnie McKenzie

and my mother Mrs. Ever Collier

Contents

Parent's/ Guardian's Foreword

There are millions of young girls; who consider sex to be a form of being loved. They've grown up with the assumption, that finding Mr. Right is the ultimate goal of a woman's life. The fairy tales are the first to introduce this theory to our daughters at a very young age; Cinderella was treated unfairly, constantly told that she'd never have or amount to anything, and was only worthy of being a servant. The magical gift of temporary possessions: escorted carriage, beautiful dress and glass slippers. Allowed Cinderella to view herself as beautiful and attract the attention of a prince. Snow White, cooked and cleaned for seven men in exchange for a place to stay, food and a sense of security. After being poisoned, only a man's kiss could restore her life. Very similar to sleeping beauty, except for a few minor details. Last but not least there's Beauty, whom gave up her freedom for her father's Trespasses. Her ultimate reward for sacrificing for a man she loved, was finding a man to love in the beast.

Our daughters are being breed with low self-esteem because of these fairy tales, the animated movies and their witnessing, the visual actions of the women in their lives, looking for a prince and yes even a beast. It is time to strengthen our daughter's self-esteem in order to stop the cycle of accepting disrespect and abuse from men. We have to assure them of controlling their own destiny. Constantly display and remind them how special and loved they are. Give them a clear understanding that love is unconditional; teach them the value of their inner beauty; so that physical actions or materialistic items won't subdue them. We can't live our daughter's lives for them, but at least by participating in unrestricted conversations, listening to their comments, explaining and allowing growth at their own pace. They will develop an assurance in the knowledge, that you are there for them and will comfort them in your arms, whenever they need you. Sometimes that knowledge along can build unbreakable self- esteem.

My husband, Mr. James Anderson

Mr. Altavis McClarin

Mrs. Minnie McKenzie

Mrs. Jillisa Lynne Jones- Craven

Mr. Jeff Shack

Ms. Lynn Moore

Ms. Neaji Kirk

You all have encouraged and inspired me.

You're becoming a woman, more with each passing day. The time has come for you, to learn the steps a young woman must take. Your body is a very special gift from God and it requires (needs) very special care.

This book is designed (made) to be a guide for you and help you to understand some of the physical (body) and emotional (feelings) changes that your body will go through as it matures (get older). Talk to your mother or an adult woman as you read this book. She has already experienced (learned about) everything that your body will go through and can give you some additional tips (help).

STEP ONE

Body Cleanliness (cleaning your body)

You should wash your hands regularly (a lot) after using the bathroom, before eating, after playing with toys and after you sneeze or cough on them. This will prevent (stop) germs from spreading. Wet your hands with warm water then rub soap on them, rub between the fingers and around your fingernails. Rinse them (rub under water) while you count to fifteen (15); this makes sure that all the germs are washed away.

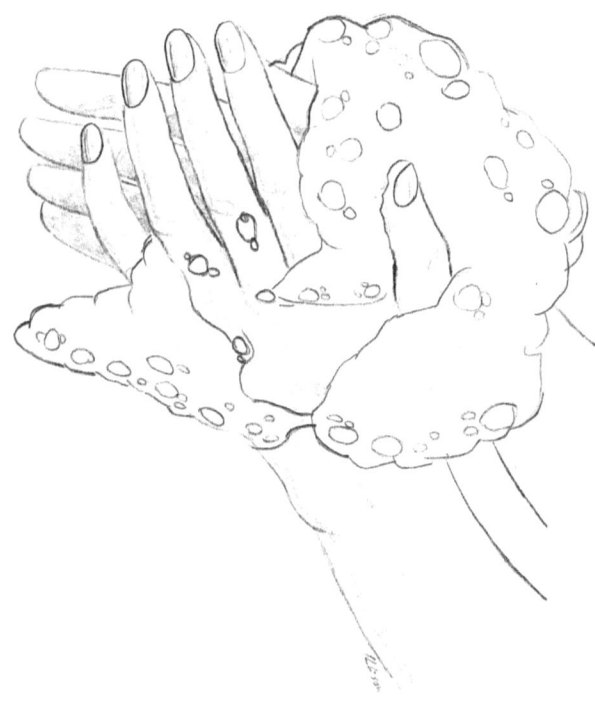

Take pride (care about it & for it) in your hair, comb it every day and brush it a lot. Your mother will use hair products (things made for hair) to style it. Short hair can be just as pretty as long hair when it is cared for.

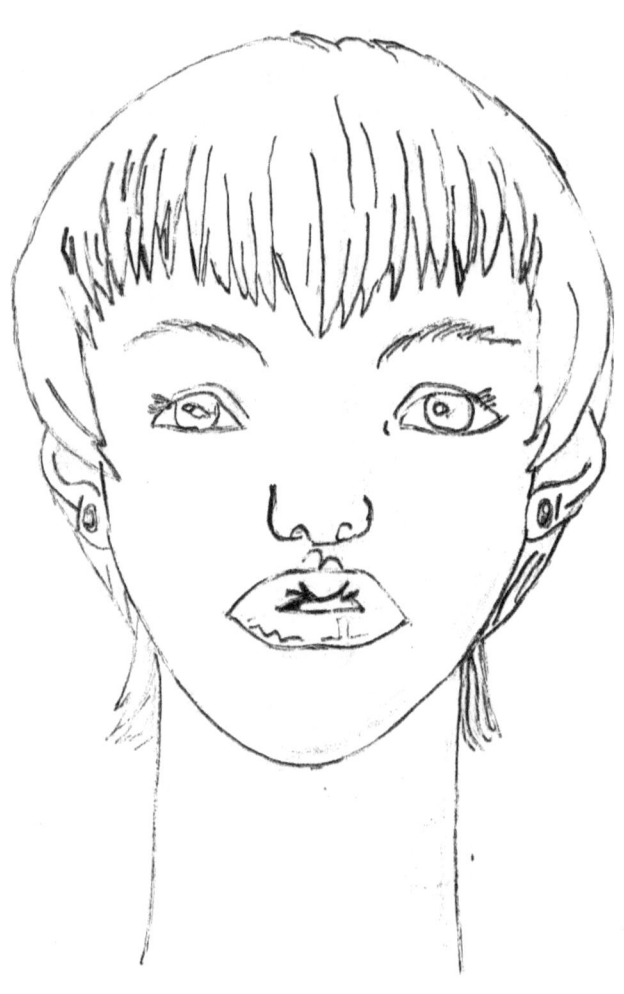

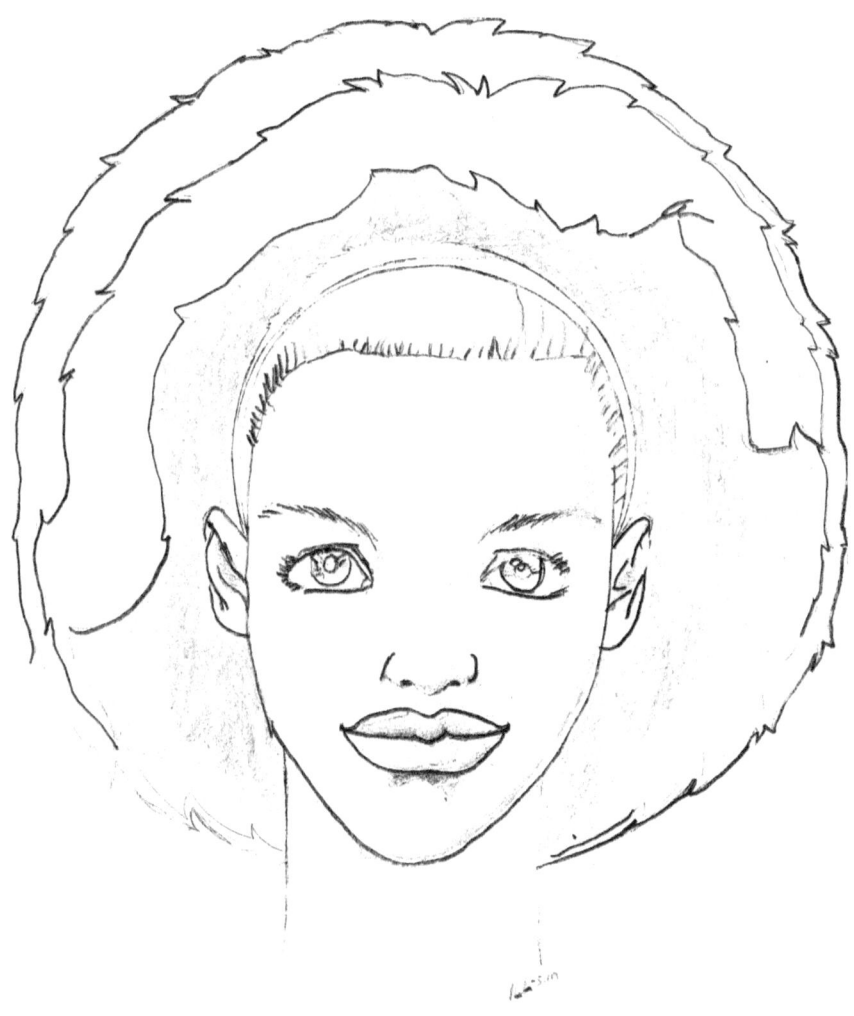

Brush your teeth every morning and every night before going to bed. This will help to keep your teeth healthy and white. Try not to eat a lot of candy; eat more fresh fruit (apples, grapes, bananas or oranges). If you don't take care of your teeth, they will began to hurt, your breath will have a bad odor (smell bad) and you may need to have false teeth as you get older.

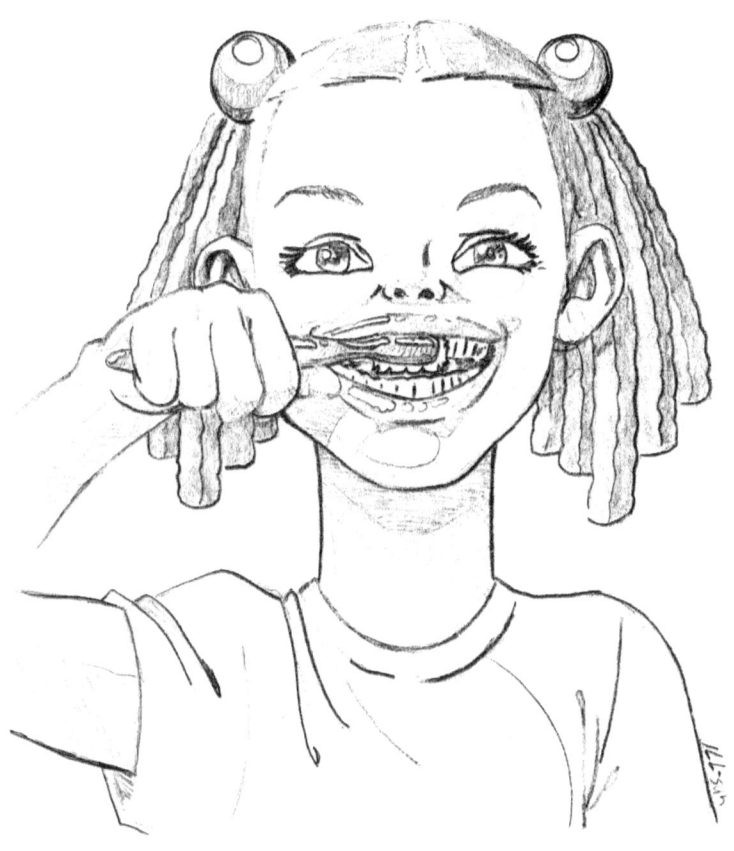

Wash your face every morning with a warm washcloth (rag), make sure you wipe the corners of your eyes to remove any of the white stuff that sometimes build up around them. Wipe behind each ear, because odors hide there; between hair washes.

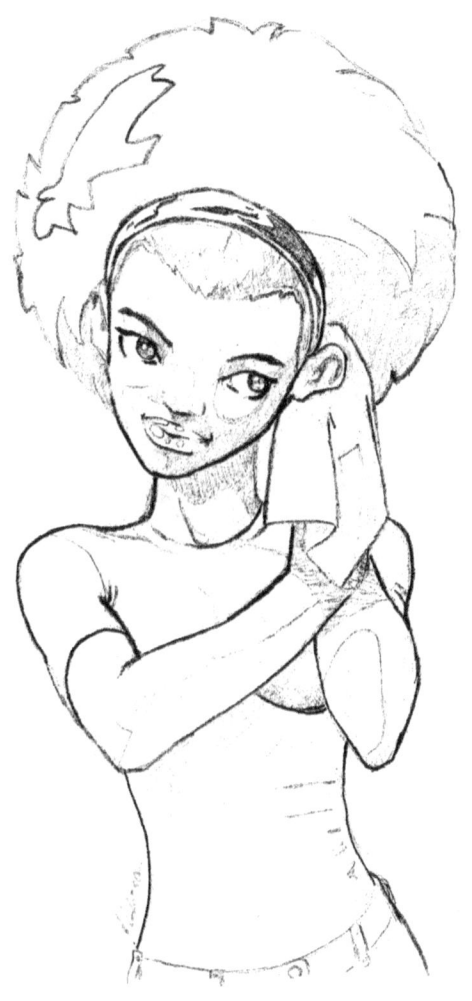

Take a bath or shower every night; because the female body, especially (most important) the vagina (tee-tee) Will have a very bad odor, if it is not properly (the right way) cleaned. When you wash your vagina (tee-tee), Don't use a lot of soap, too much soap will make it sting (hurt).

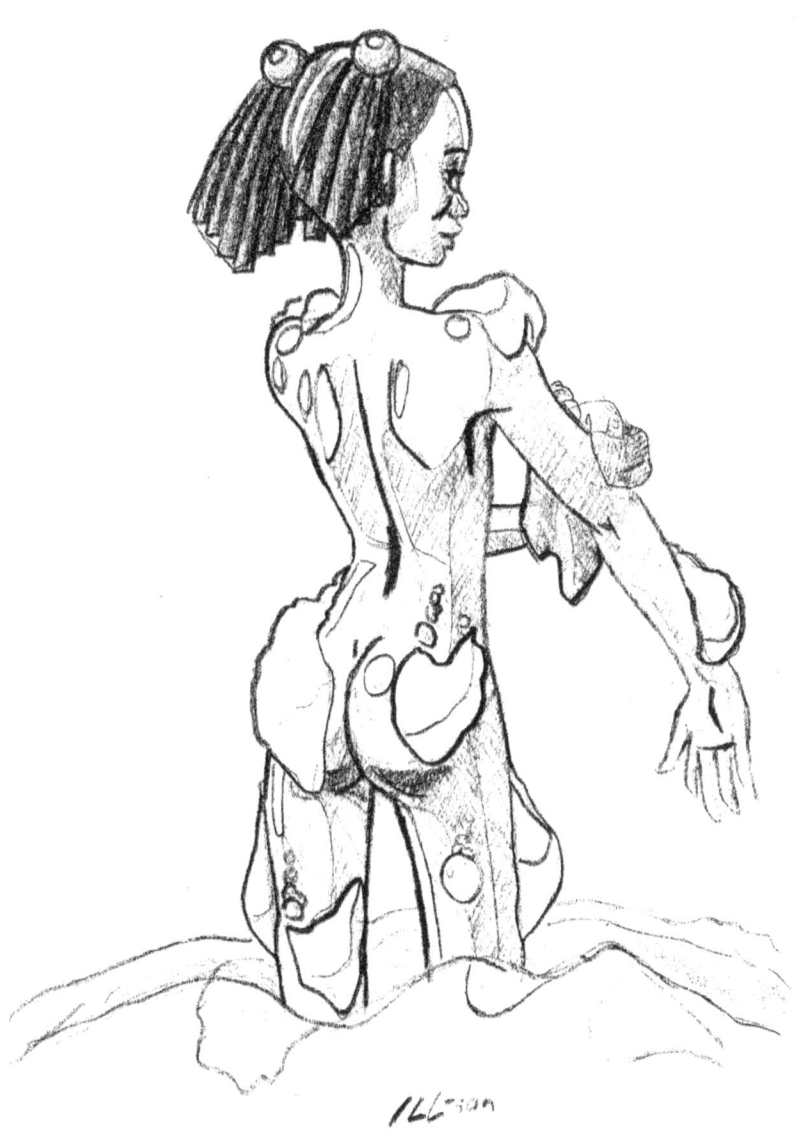

Wear clean panties every day, because germs can travel (move around) on clothing. Each time after you urinate (tee-tee), wipe from the front of your vagina toward the back. This will help keep germs from passing to the vagina. Wash your hands when finished, with soap and warm water. If you have a bowel movement (boo-boo or #2) wipe from the bottom up to the back. Wash your hands (with soap and warm water).

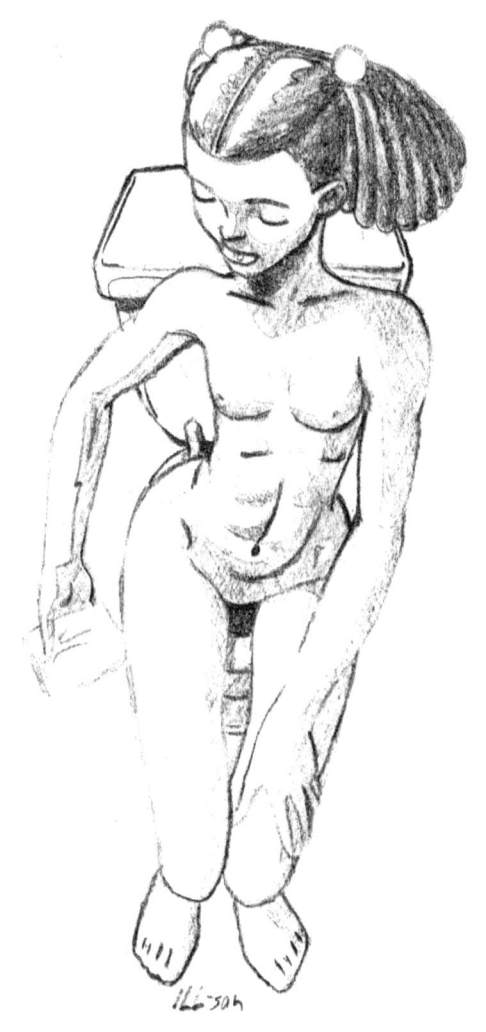

STEP TWO

Body Responsibility
(taking care of your body)

Get eight hours or more of sleep every night; a rested body is strong, alert and can think clearly.

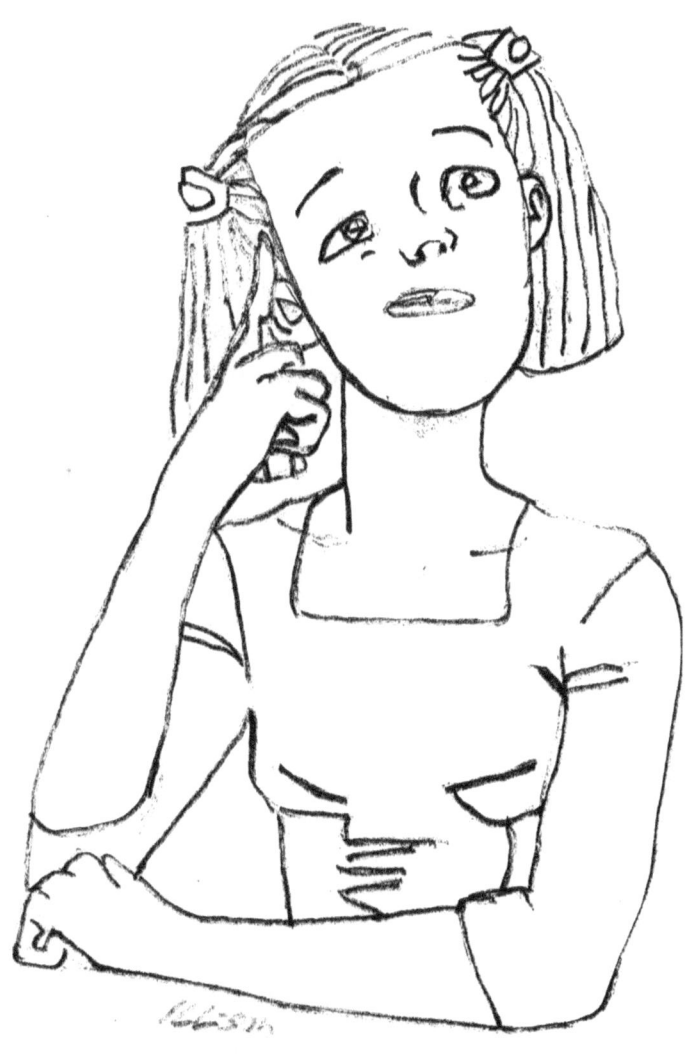

A tired body can't think clearly, has a hard time sitting up straight and can't focus on anything. Drink water every day and try not to drink too many sodas. Too much acidity (something in sodas) will cause urinary (tee-tee) Problems. Drinking water is good for your body.

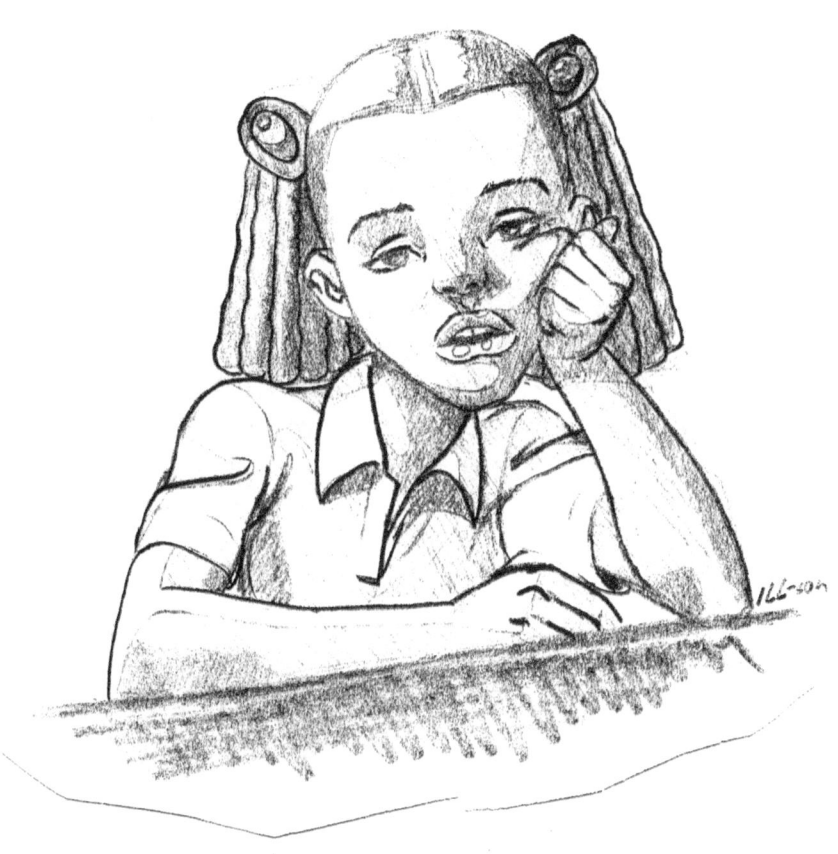

Don't take prescription drugs (pills with someone else name) unless your name is on them, an adult or parent should supervise (give them to you) when you need to take it.

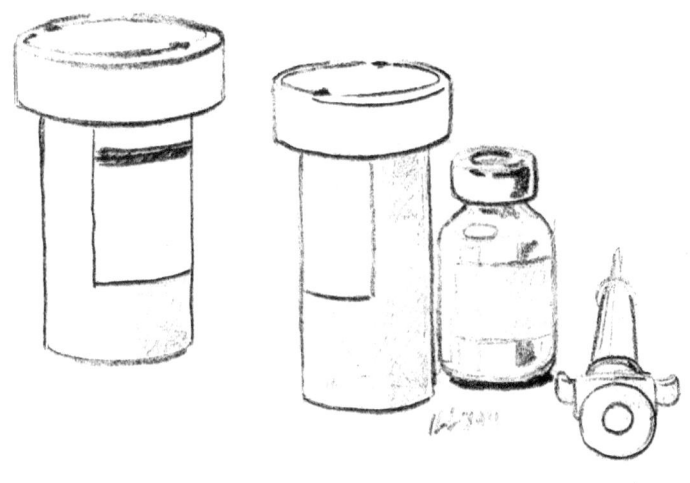

Don't take street drugs (drugs being given to you free or sold to you). It is very important that you don't experiment (try or test) with drugs, it is usually the first try that gets your body addicted. Addiction to a drug, will make you do anything to get it; you won't care about how you look, smell, who you have to hurt or steal from, to get drugs and it could kill you.

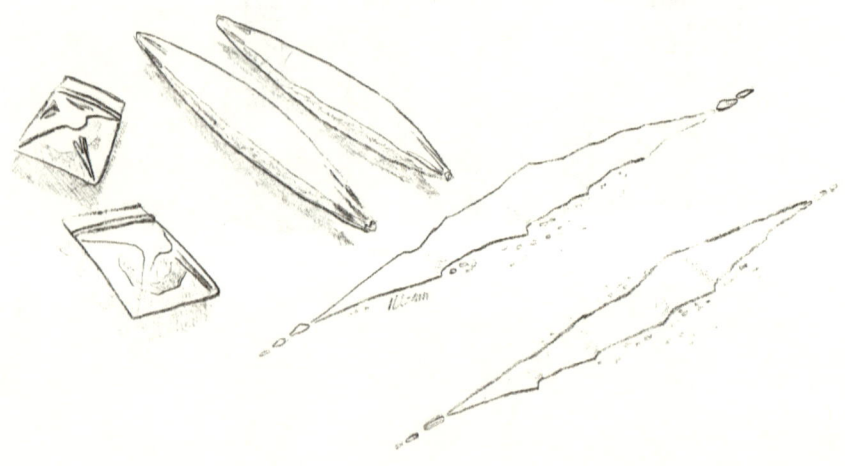

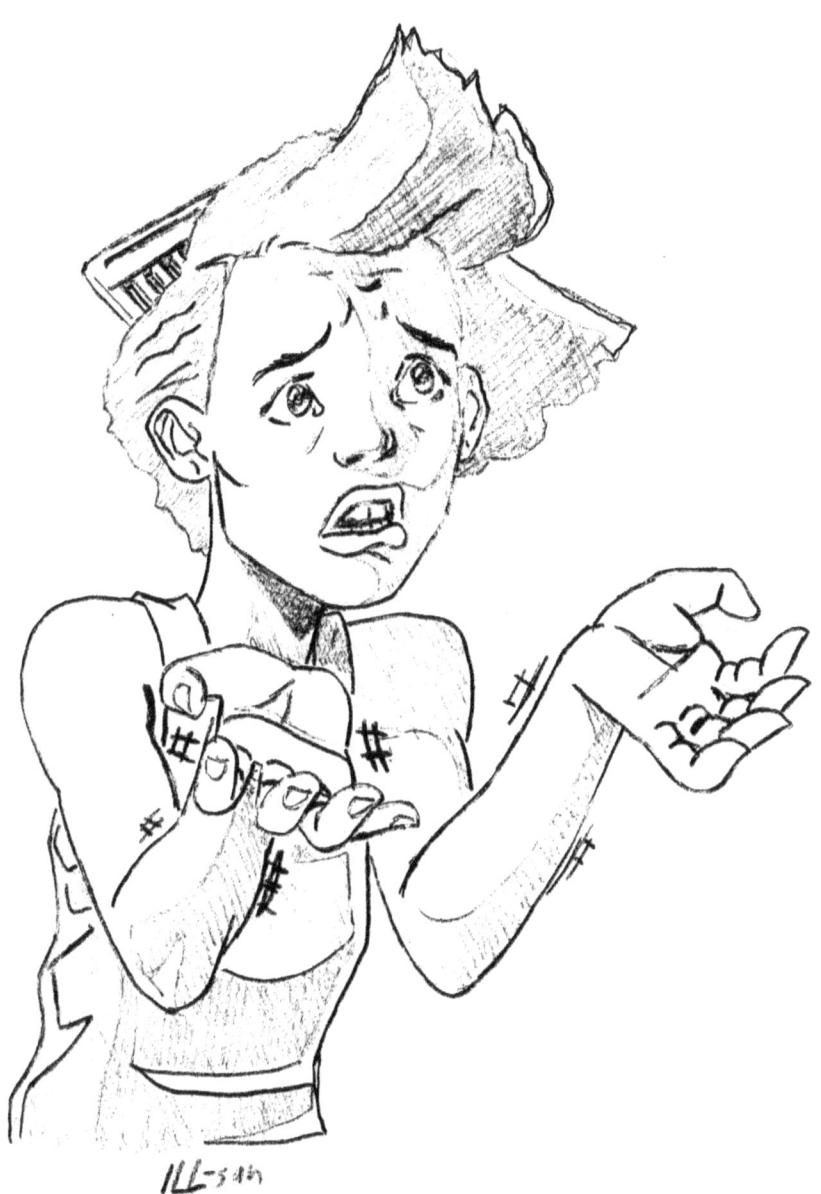

Don't ever try smoking; it doesn't make you look cool. It's easy to start, but very hard to stop. Cigarettes can cause a lot of different illnesses (sickness) especially breathing problems.

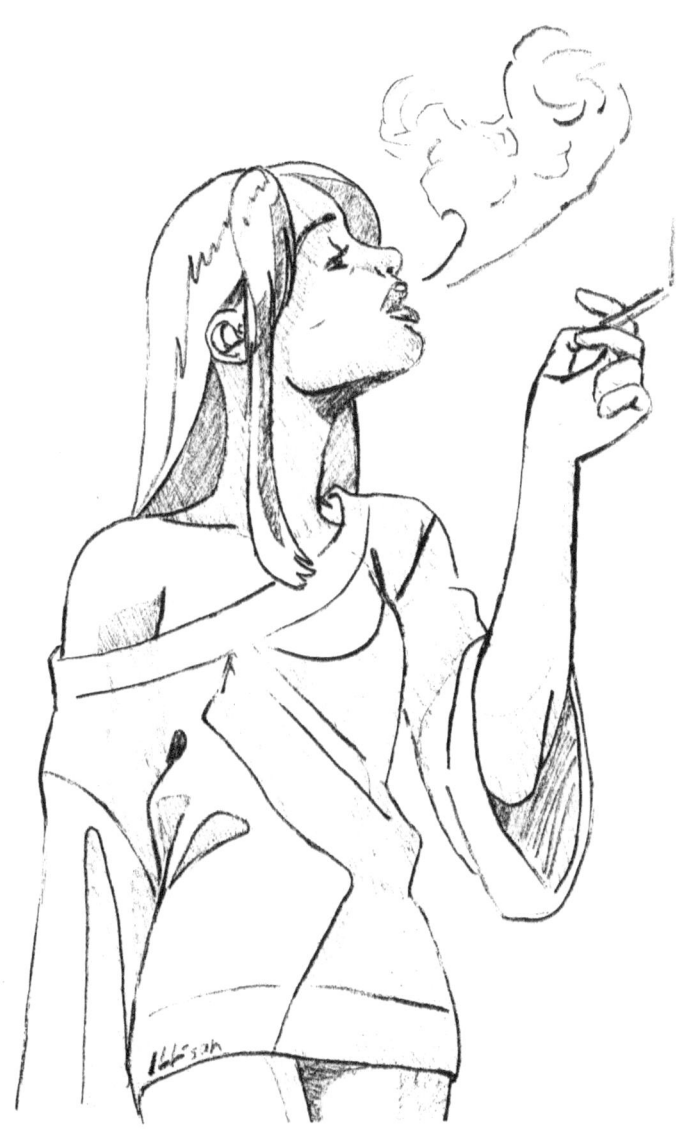

Don't drink beer, wine or liquor. You are too young to make these decisions now. Wait until You become 21 years old and decide for yourself, not because someone you know does it. Take care of your body and it will take care of you, by being strong and healthy.

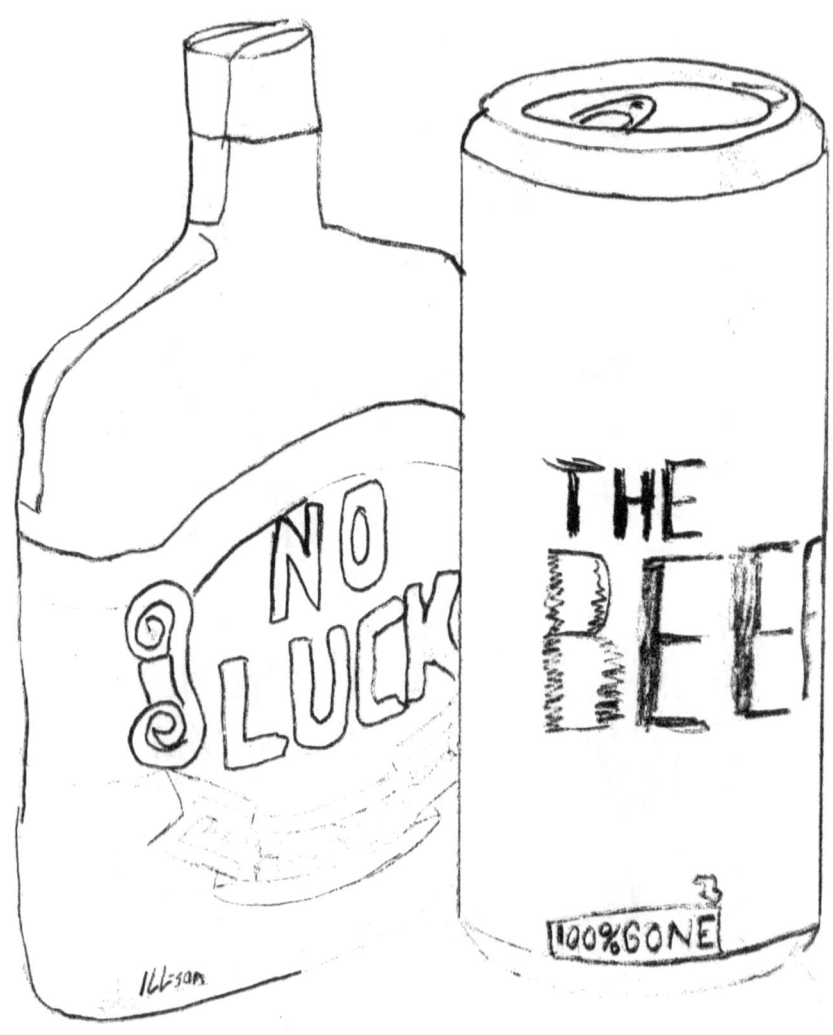

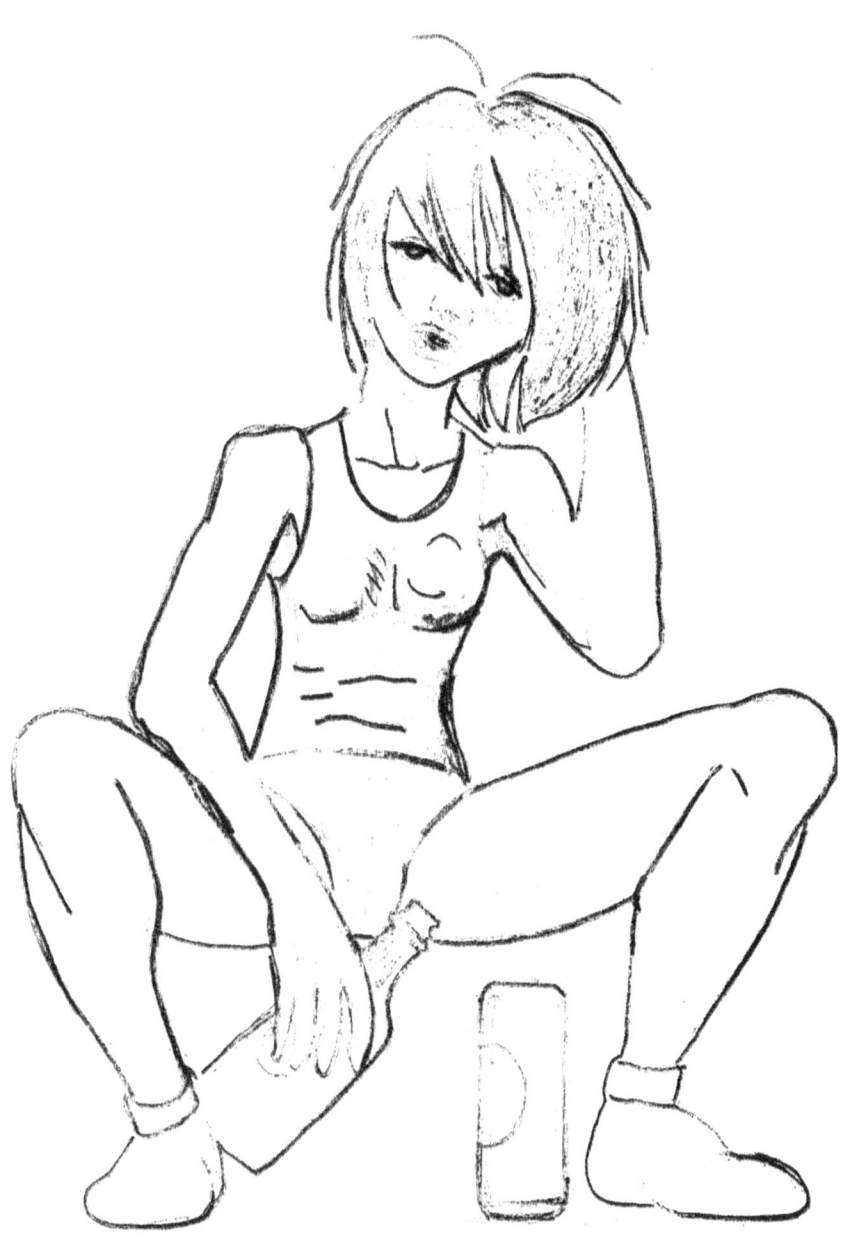

Don't sniff paint, glue, gas or cleaning chemicals. This will affect your breathing and your brain. It could also kill you.

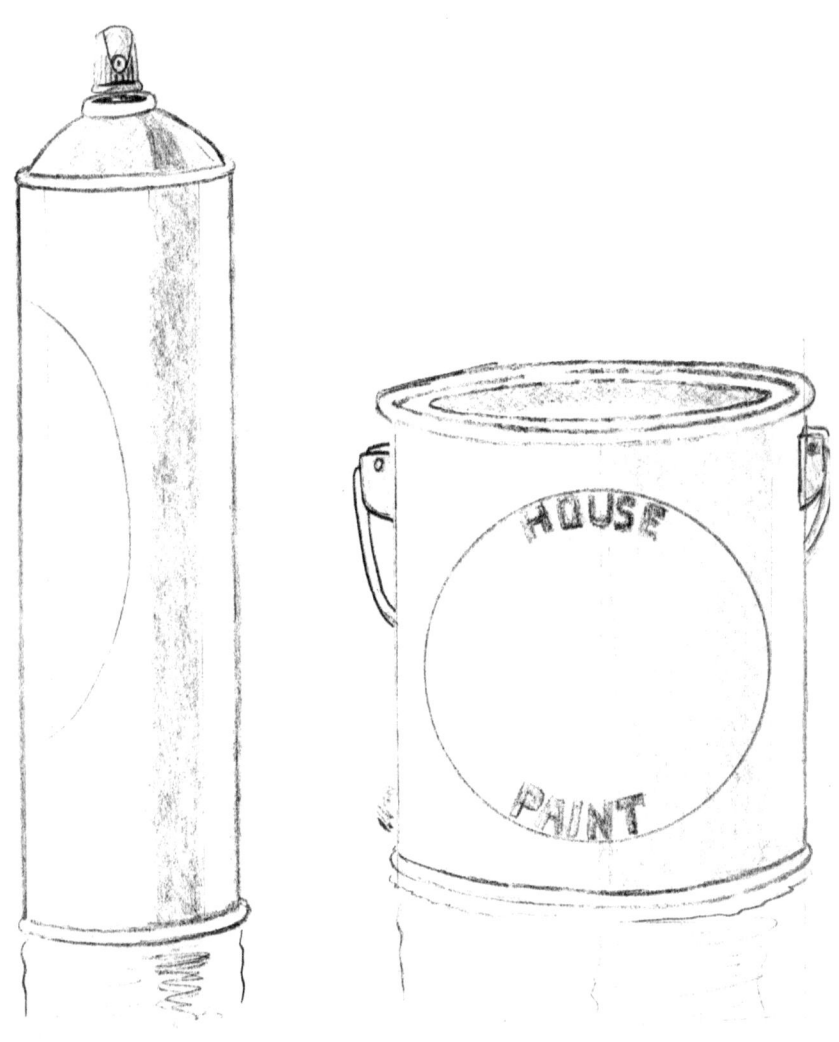

Before getting a tattoo (word or picture placed on the skin), think about all the steps involved, ask an adult and you questions. Tattoos are placed on the skin with needles; if an infection (pain, swelling blood and pus) starts there is a risk to your health. If you change your mind later, it is very expensive to remove.

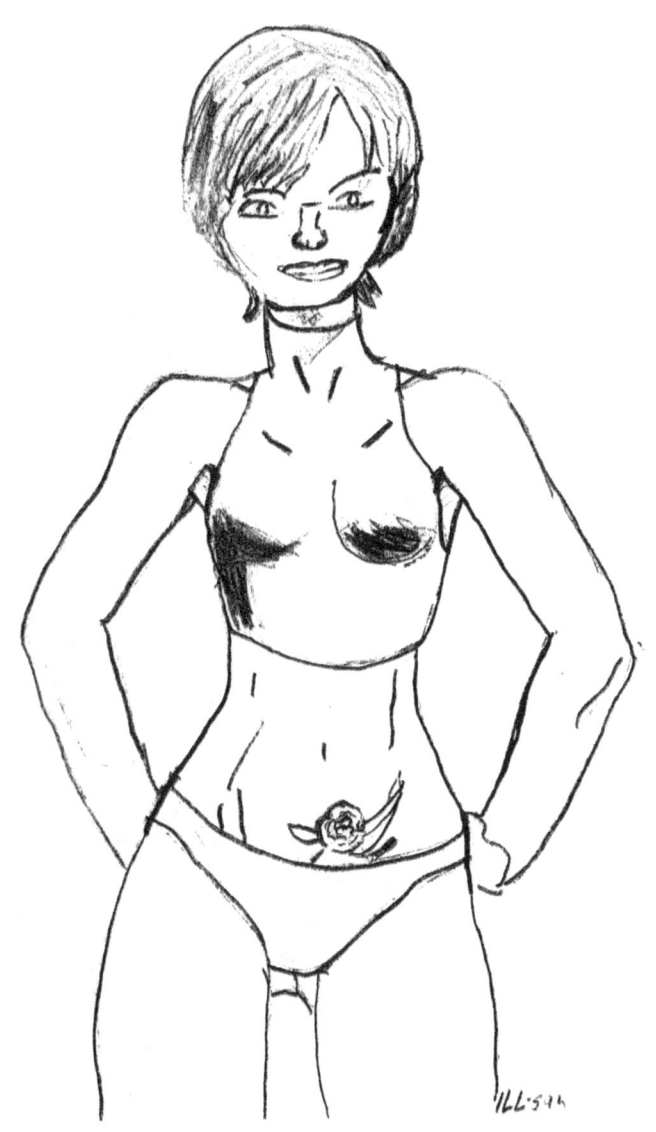

Don't write on your skin with an ink pen or marker. It could cause problems with your skin.

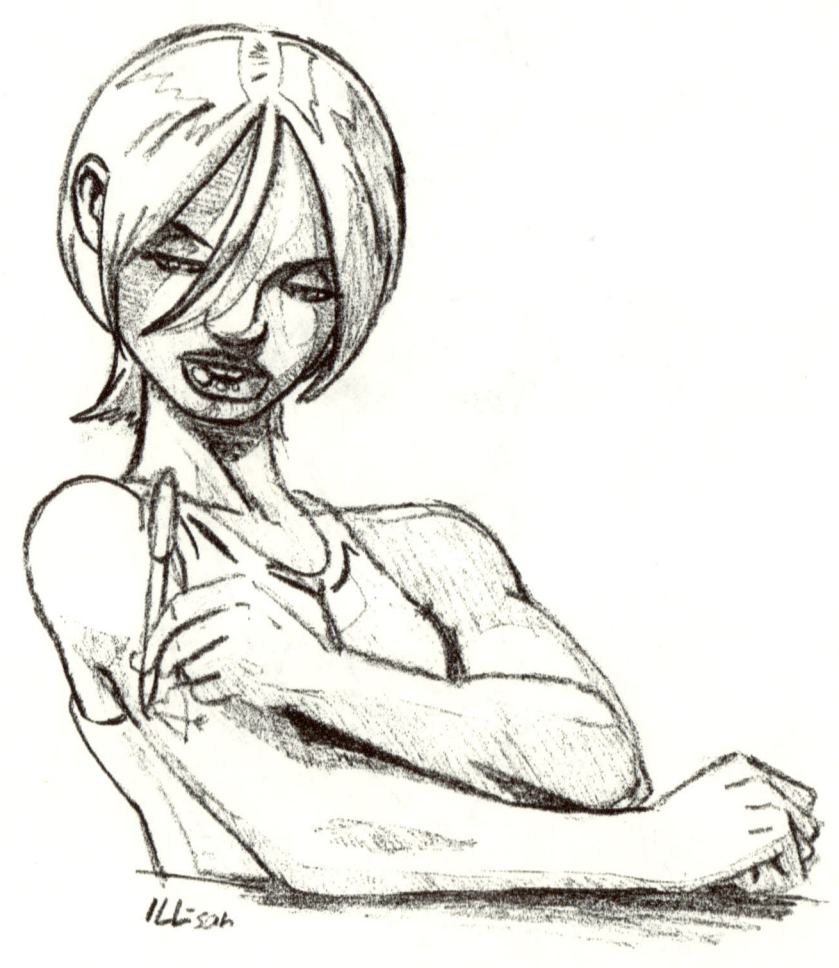

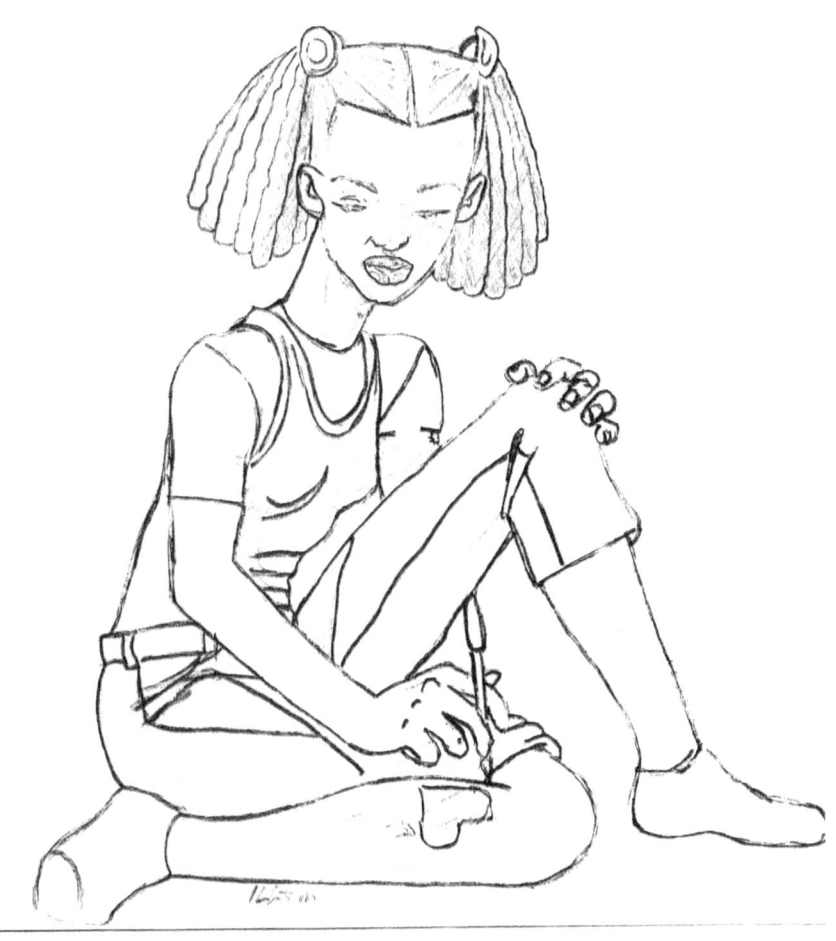

STEP THREE
Mentality (way of thinking)

Most boys are nice and say nice things about you, when you first meet them. Get to Know him by talking to him and listening to him. His real personality (naughty or nice) will be revealed (shown) in his actions (the way he acts) and words (what he says). If he refers (speak of) To girls as ugly or nasty names, he doesn't respect women and will say the same thing about you.

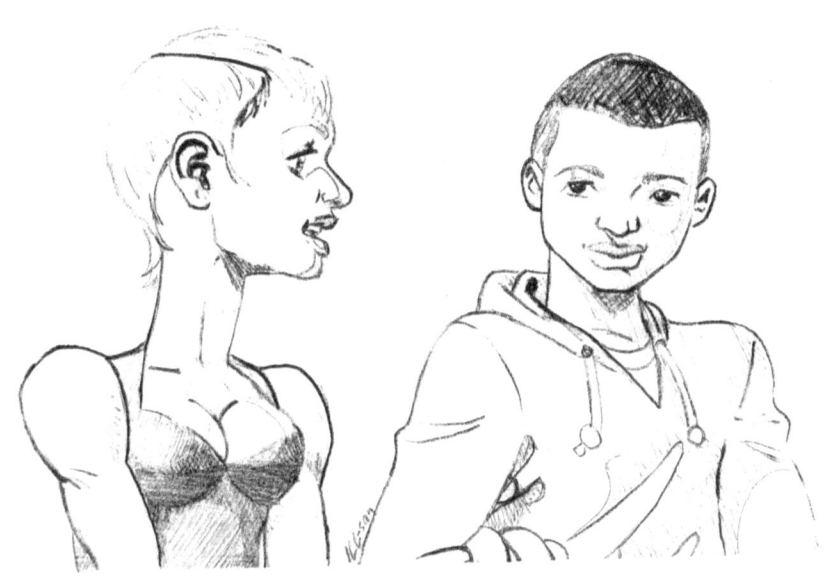

Don't allow a boy to disrespect you by cursing or calling you nasty names. You can do this by Leaving the crowd when he walks up. Report his nasty language and actions to a teacher or adult. Make sure that you also tell your parents, they will follow up (talk about the problem) with the teacher or adult and his parents. If you don't do anything about his actions he will get worst. Don't be afraid to tell, he only controls (has power over) what you give him.

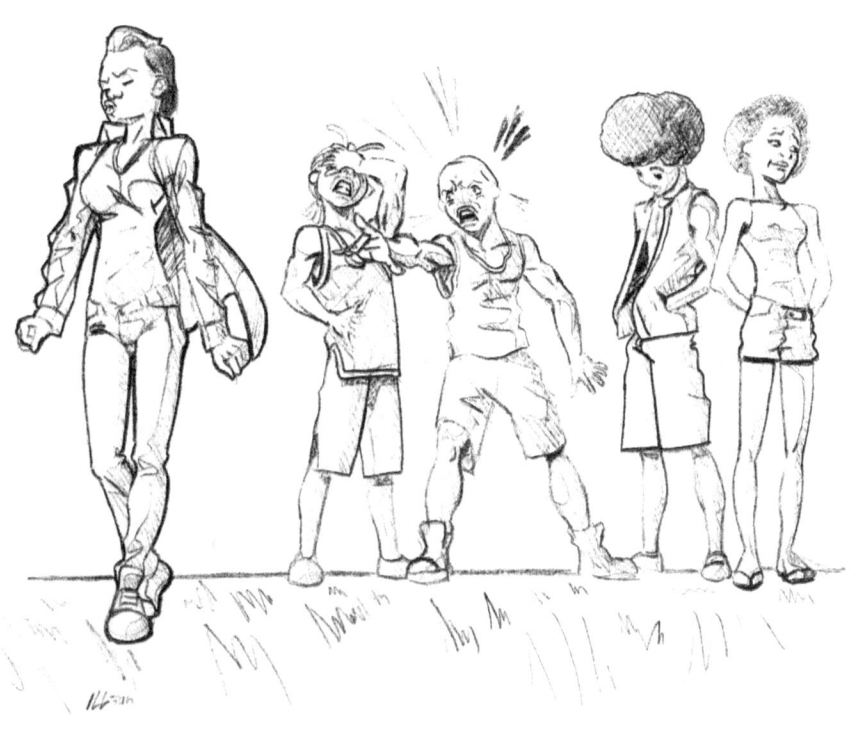

A boy should value (listen to) what you say and think. He doesn't have to agree with it, but he Should respect (allow you to speak) your ability to think and rationalize (have a thought and explain). If a boy likes you, he'll respect you; he won't force you to do anything. There is no right or wrong, when it concerns (comes from) anyone's personal opinion (thoughts or beliefs), we all have to practice more on respecting each other's thoughts; whether we agree with it or not.

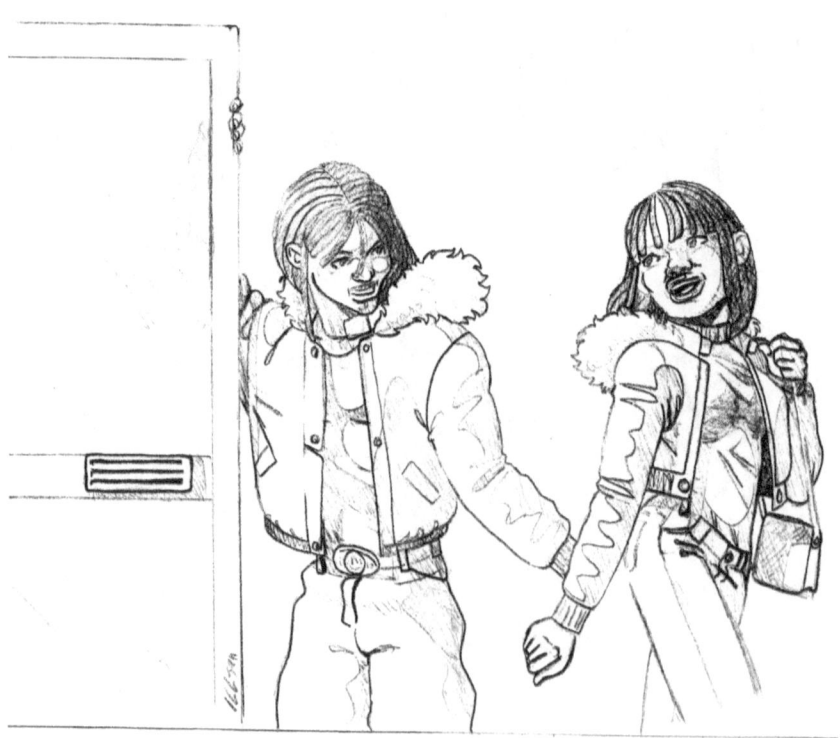

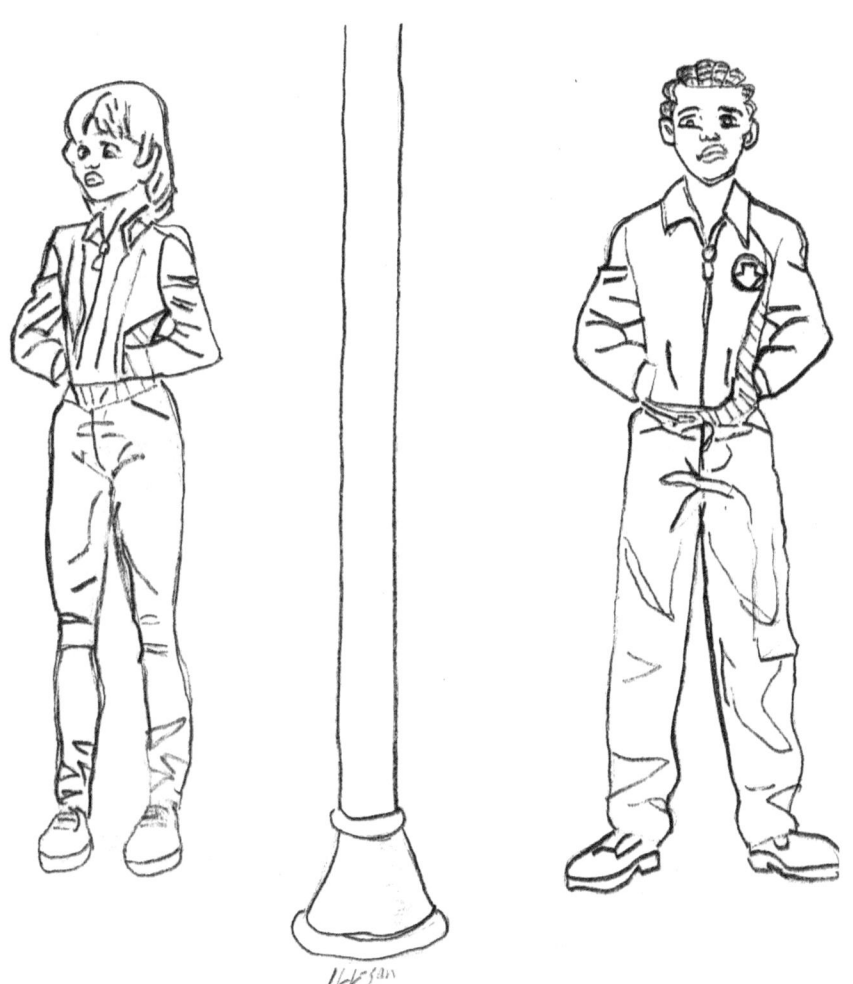

People should like you, for who you are, if you have to act to get someone to like you, you will change into what they want you to be. Don't ever <u>not</u> be yourself. If the person is worth having, as a friend, they will be a friend. If you always have to do something for them, in order to be their friend, they could never be a good friend to you.

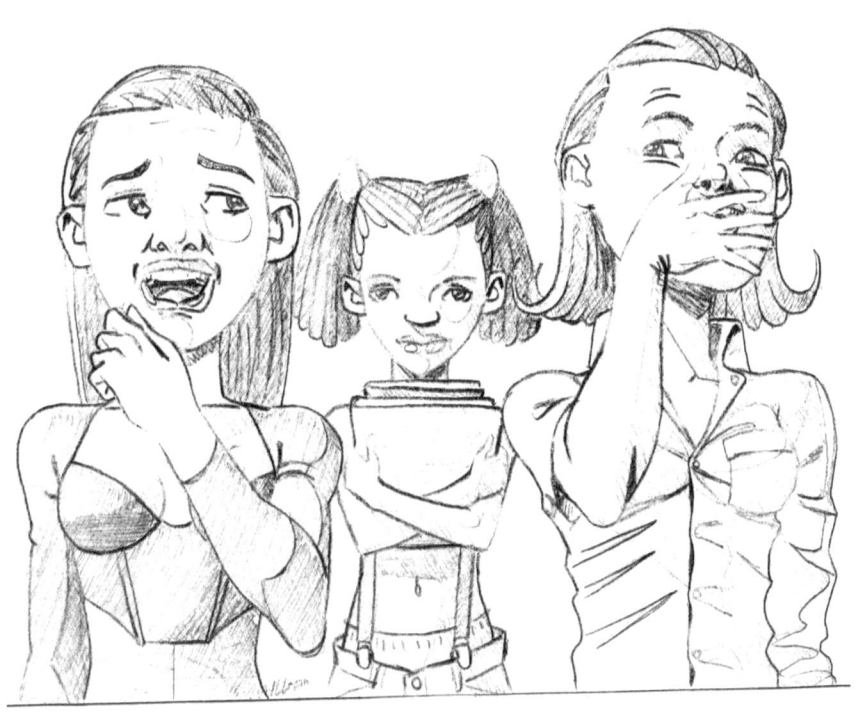

Being beautiful involves (is about) more than just looks, size, hair, and race (color). Beauty is displayed (seen) in your actions (what you do or say and how you do or say something). Look at yourself and answer the following questions truthfully.

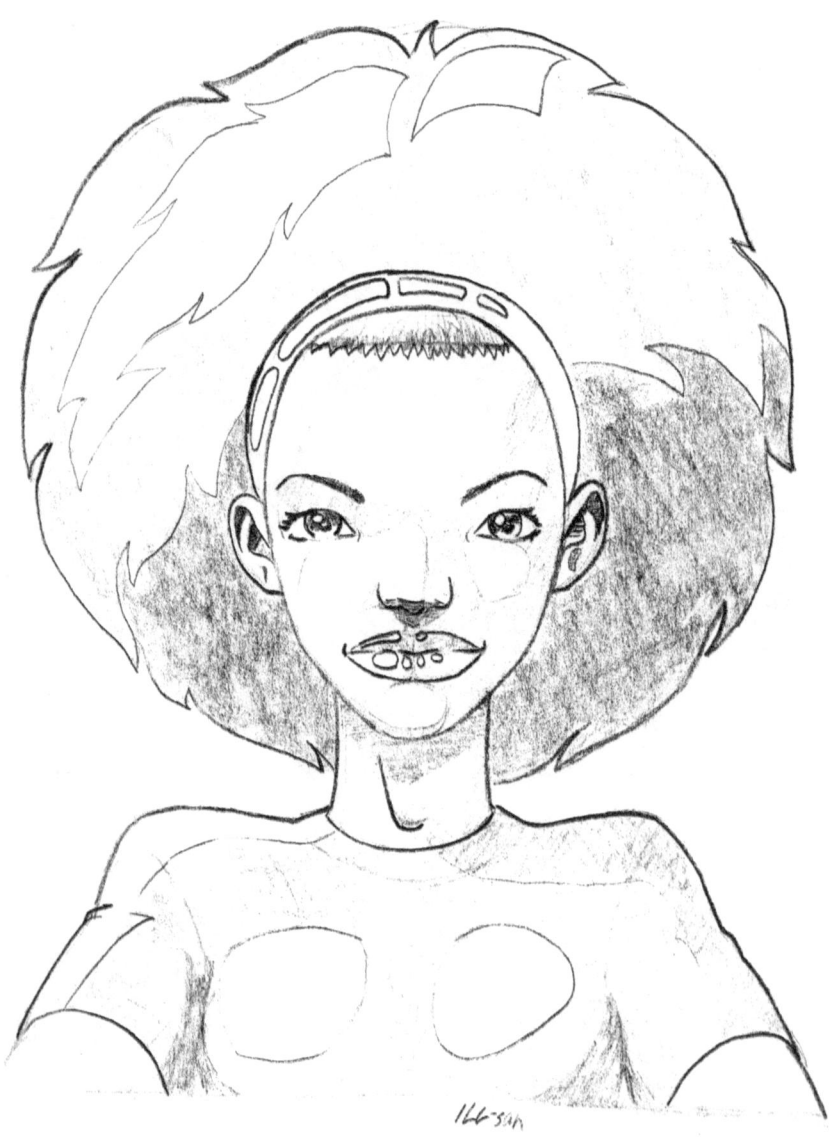

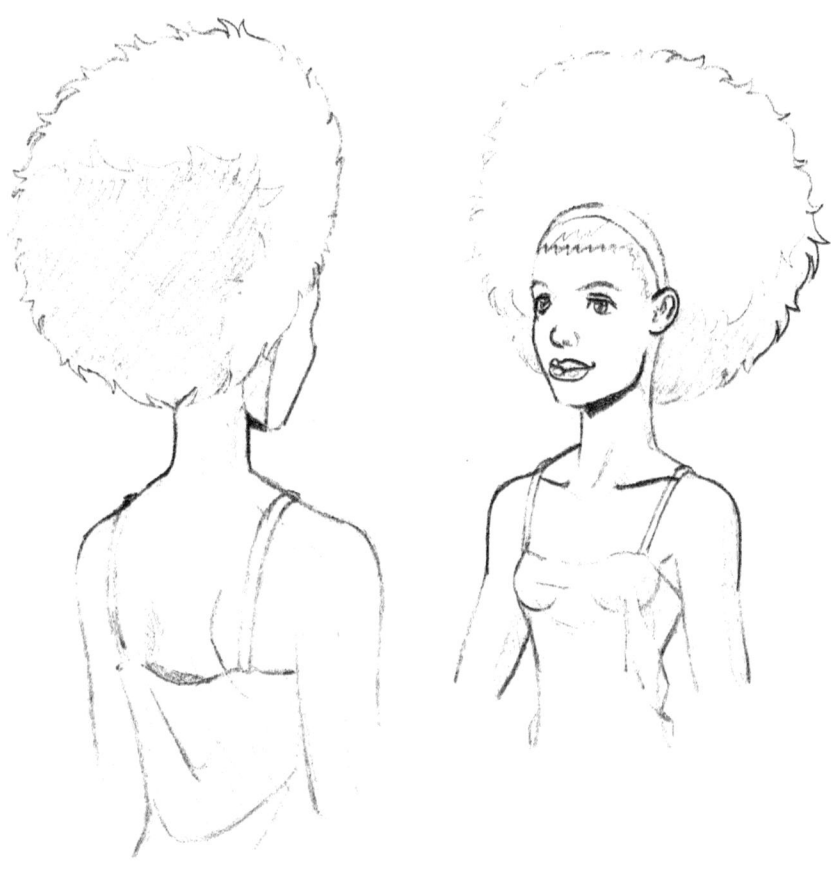

Do you respect yourself and others? Do you treat people with respect or treat them bad to impress someone.

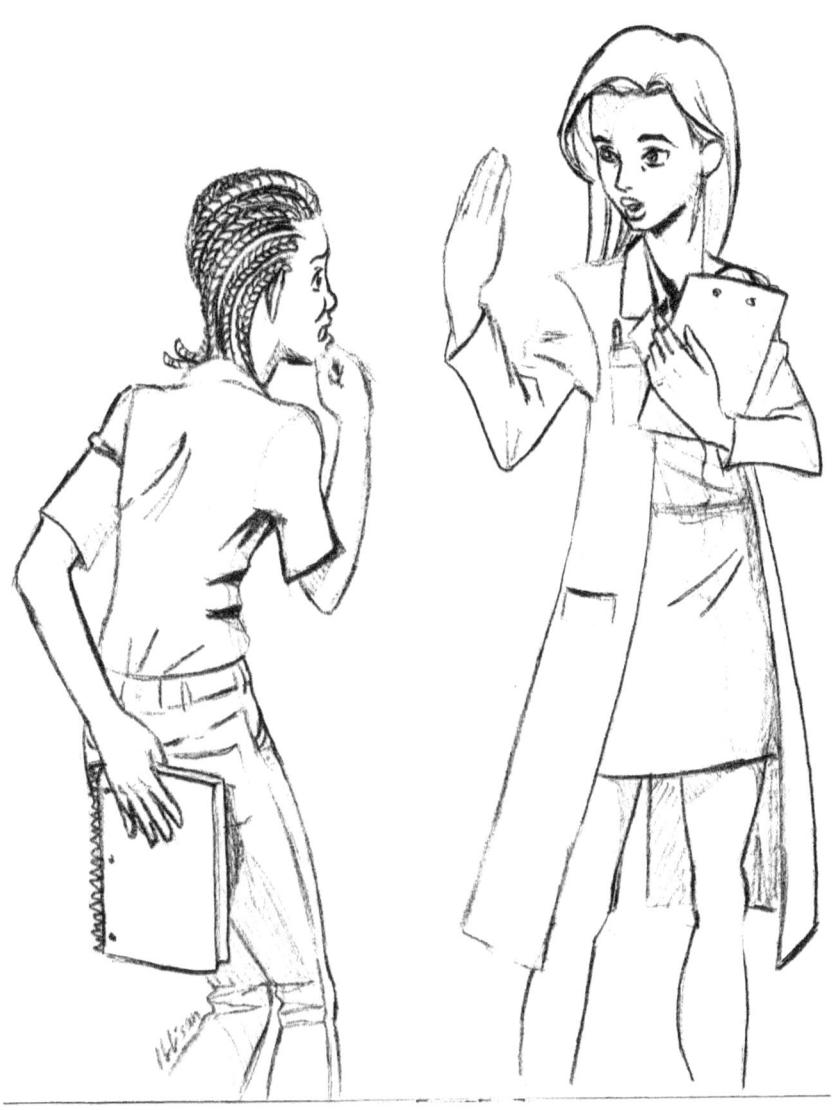

Can you control your attitude? If someone doesn't do what you expect or want them to, how do you act?

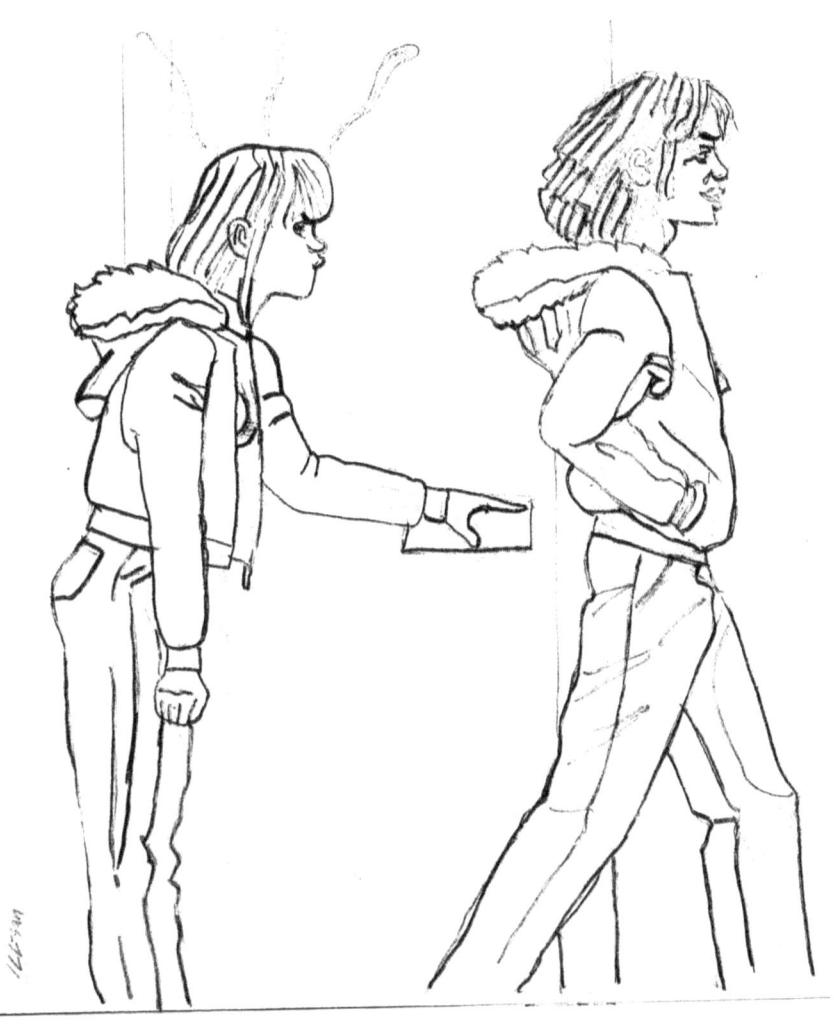

Do you do think first then act? Think about what you're trying to do first, think of different ways to do it, then pick an option (choices) and try it.

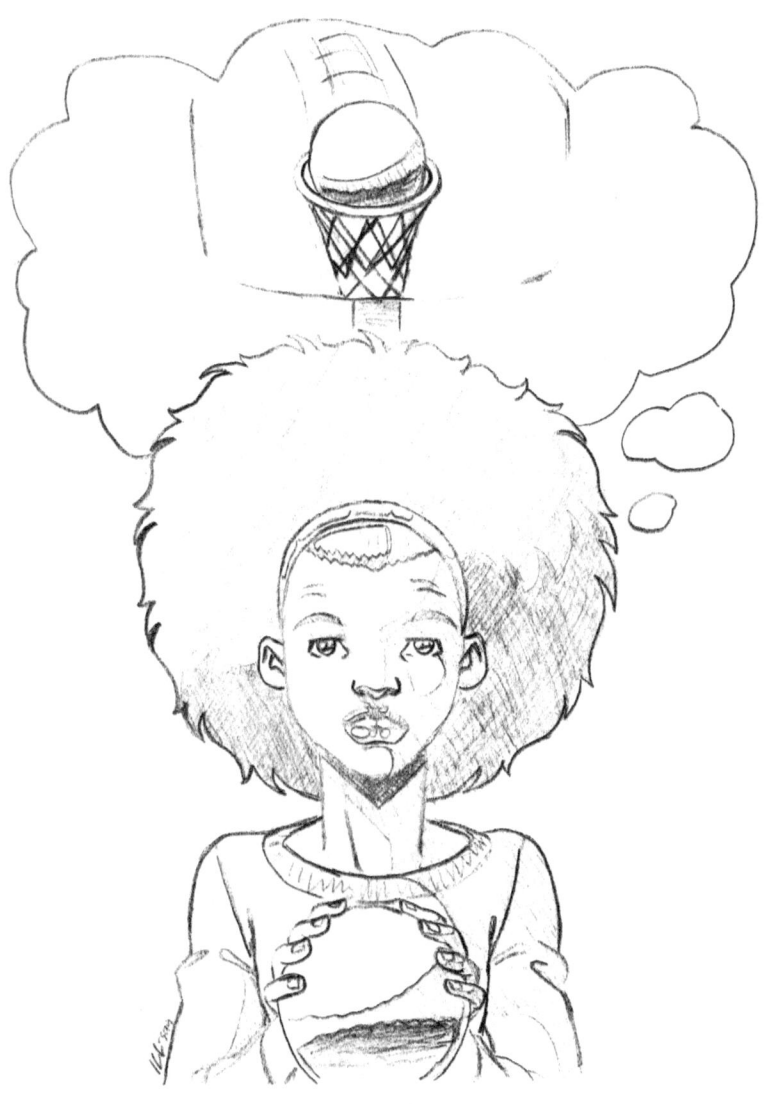

Do you think for yourself? Do you walk, talk, dress and act like a young lady?

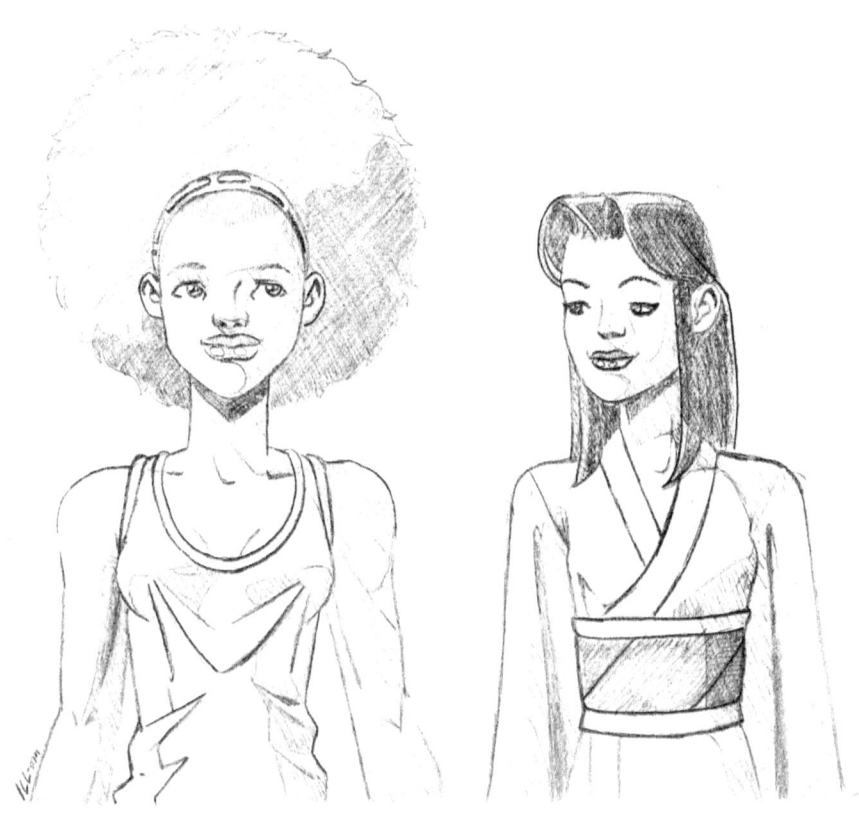

If you said or thought no to any of these questions, then work on it. It takes practice. Control your attitude; never act out in anger; count to ten, then think before you act. Never do something that you know is wrong or questionable (you're not sure about) just Because everyone else is doing it. Trust yourself, if it doesn't feel right, it is not right for you; walk away. Always think for yourself.

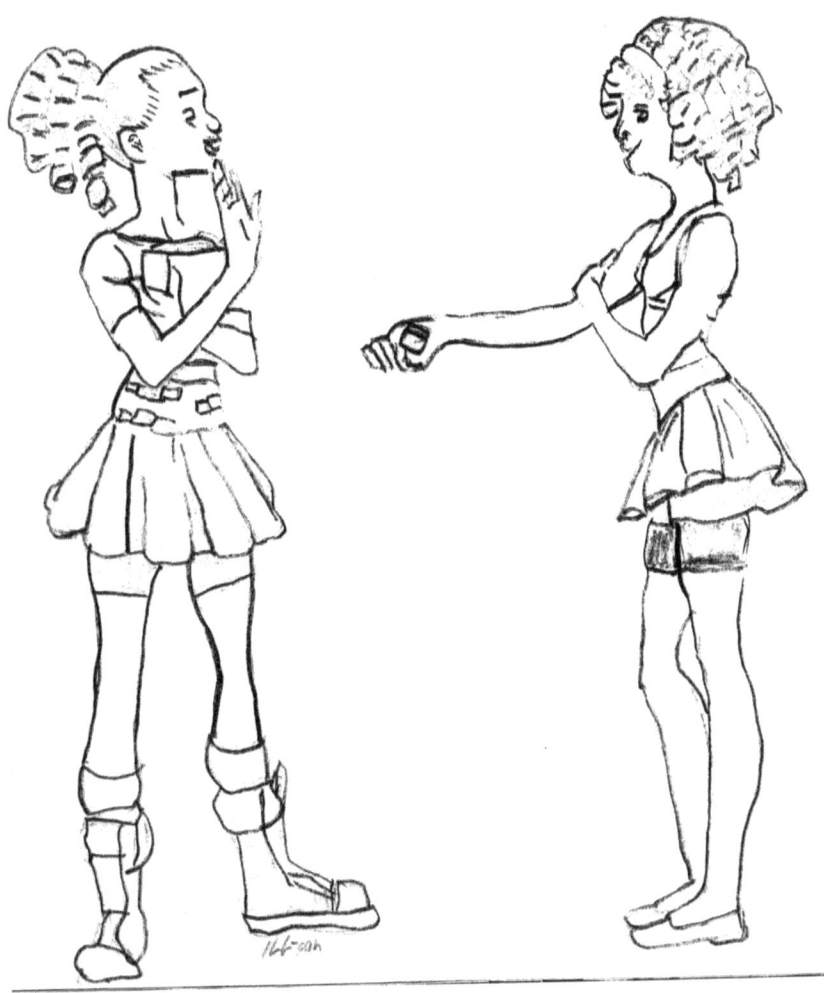

Practice making your own decisions: Start with simple things like what to wear, eat or drink discuss (Talk about) your choices with your mom or an adult; this trains you to think and rationalize (explain and understand you reasoning (why)). If something doesn't seem right or you don't understand it; talk to your mom or an adult woman. They were once your age and can guide or help you make decisions.

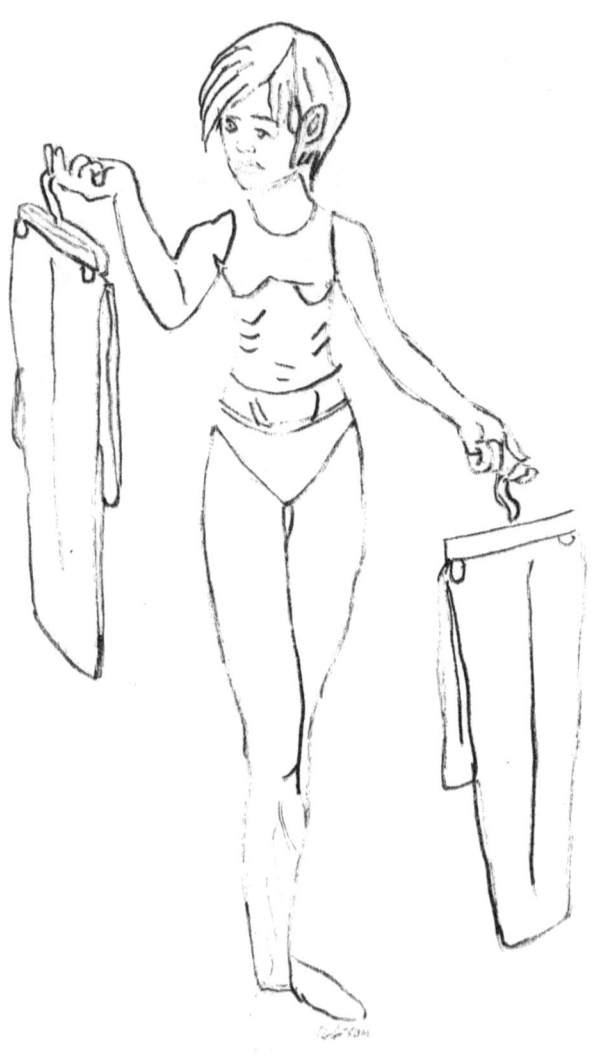

When you practice making decisions about what to wear use rules (guidelines).Rules are made to safeguard you. I know that some rules seem hard to follow, but by practicing your decision making, following rules will become easier. You will begin to understand the reasons for the rules.

For school, church, parties and special events (weddings or programs) you need to dress really nice. Don't wear tight clothes; dirty clothes, clothes with holes in them, clothes that show too much of your body, or clothes that are too big.

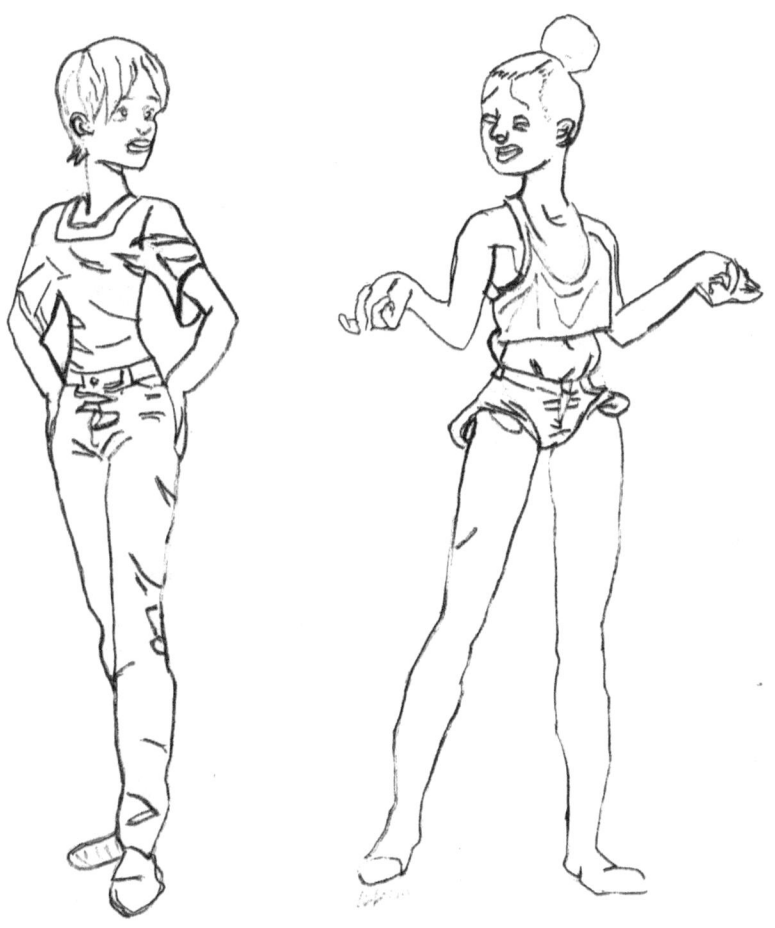

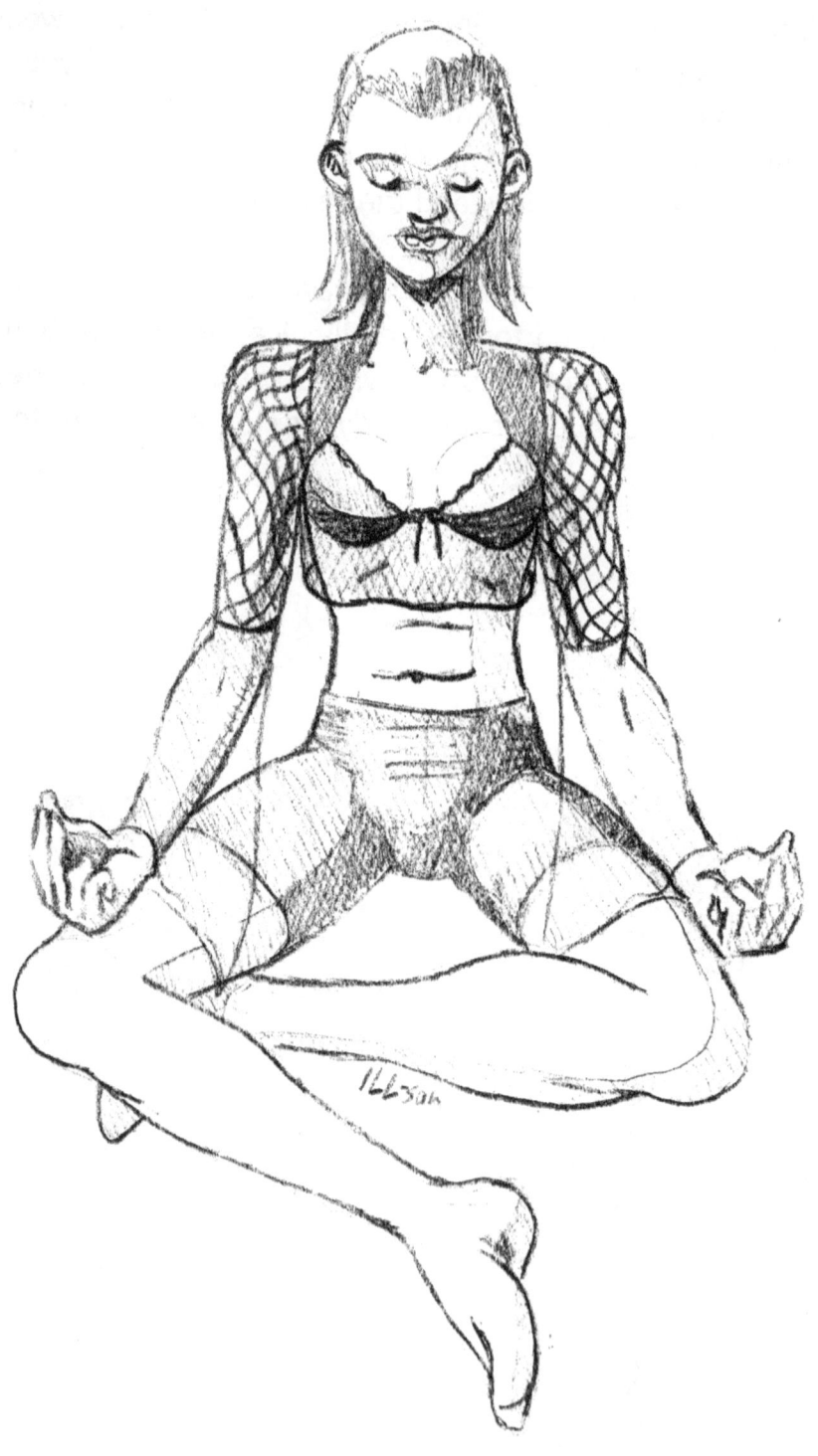

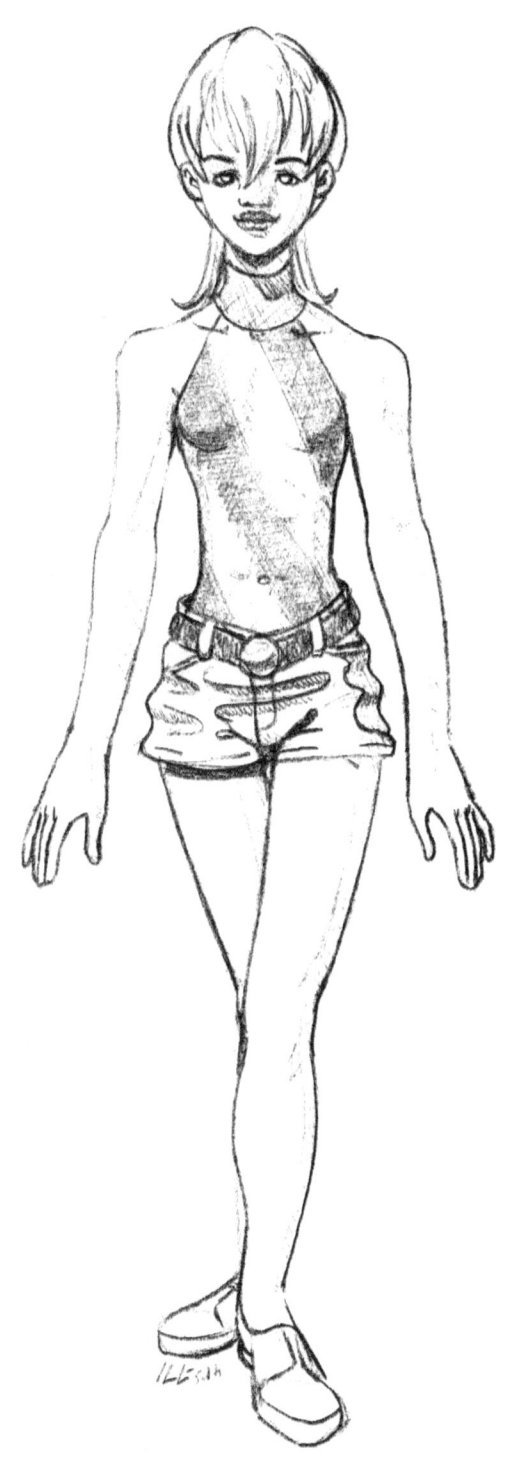

Speak softly and clearly pronounce your words. Never yell, curse or talk nasty to Show off. People will only respect you; when you respect yourself. When in school pay close attention to the teacher's lesson and study all of your assignments (homework).

Teachers have made a decision to live their life; helping you prepare (get ready) to live Your life with the right tools (education). Every subject (math, reading, science and history) is a tool, which you will need in life to help making decisions.

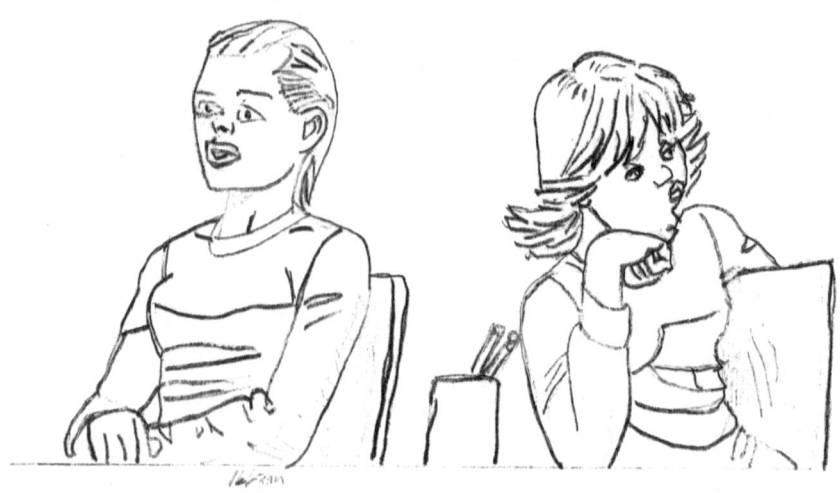

No one is perfect, we all make mistakes, learn from them (mistakes). Look at every step that lead to the mistake and try to figure how to improve it the next time.

Practicing this step will help you prevent (stop) repeating the same mistakes. Don't blame others for your mistakes; always tell the truth, even if the truth might get You or someone else in trouble.

If a person ask you to lie for them; don't do it, because a lie will grow and cause innocent people to be hurt. If you lie for them; one day, they may tell a lie on you.

Always be honest (tell the truth) with yourself and others. People will respect and trust you. This practice will also help you learn, to trust and respect yourself. If you don't respect yourself, no one will respect you. Respect is earned; not given,

STEP FOUR

Body Protection (protecting your body)

No girl or boy should ever hit you; for any reason. If they do get away from them and tell an adult what happened. Walking away from someone who hit you, does not make you a scary cat. Fighting someone who hit you does not make you brave or a hero. A true friend would never hurt you, make fun of you or ask you to do something wrong.

Don't believe everything that someone tells you, because some kids and some adults like to trick you, hurt you or impress (make you like them) you by lying. Remember to practice thinking for yourself and always think before you act.

It is safe to say hello to a stranger; but never go anywhere with a stranger, without your parents' permission. Don't go into anyone's house or let anyone into your house until your parents say it is alright to do. if a stranger in a car tries to show or give you something; Don't get close to them. Back away , so they can't grab you. Walk away as quickly as you can.

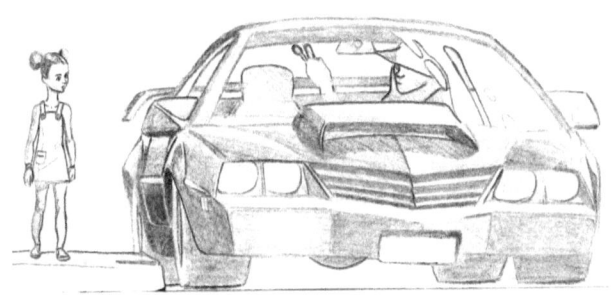

If someone hurts you; scares you, or does something to you, that you know is wrong. Tell your parents or an adult you trust (you know that you are safe with them). A policeman or a policewoman will help keep you safe.

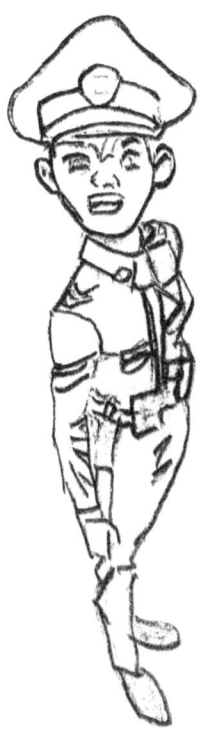
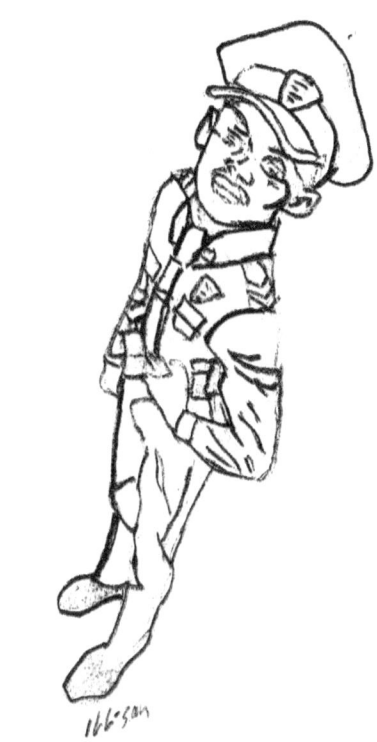

A store is the safest place to get help when you are lost or afraid. If you go to a store. Talk to the person behind the counter and ask them to call the police for help.

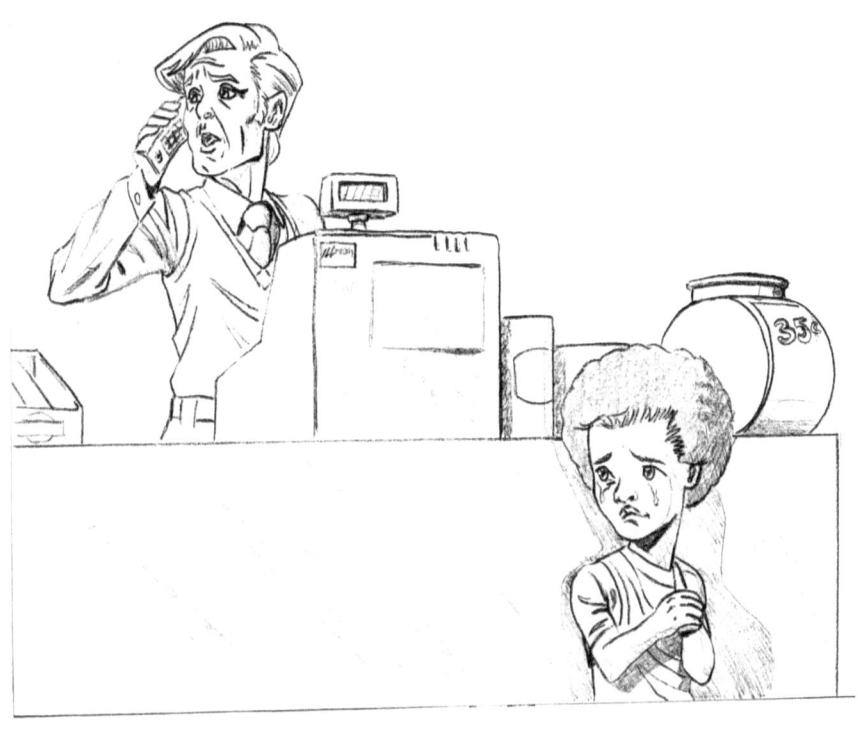

STEP FIVE
Puberty (body changes)

Puberty is a word used to describe the changes a male or female body goes through. You will begin to have very strong emotions (happiness, sadness) without any reason.

As your body starts to develop (change) it begins the process of Puberty. Puberty is: a point(certain time) in a girl's life where she can become pregnant or a point (certain time) in a boy's life, where he can make a girl pregnant.

You can only become pregnant (have a baby) by having sexual intercourse (sex) with a boy or man. Sex is a precious gift; that God gave men and women, for the purpose of creating a family, while sharing life, love and trust, as husband and wife.

Sometimes people use this gift for their own reasons. If you have questions about sex, please talk to your mom or an adult you love and trust. Young people, even teenagers may not be able to answer your questions, with the truth and Delicacy (right way) needed for you. You are very special and I don't want you to be misled (lied to or given the wrong information).

Think before you act

Sex is not; something you do, just to show someone you like them. Sex is not; being loved nor giving love. Sex is not; something you do, in order to make a boy or man like or love you. Sex is not; a weapon for a woman or a man to use against anyone. Sex is not; a way to party. Sex is not; love.

Think for yourself, no one can make these life decisions for you. Always think before you act, ask yourself questions. You won't always make the right decisions, but you'll learn and grow from your mistakes. Remember; you have to review the mistakes, in order to prevent (not make) the same mistakes.

As your body grows, the two small tips on your chest will become breast. Your mom can help you decide, when you'll need a training bra. A training bra is used to teach you how to wear a bra and to cover your breast. Training bras are flat, come in different colors and are sized by your chest.

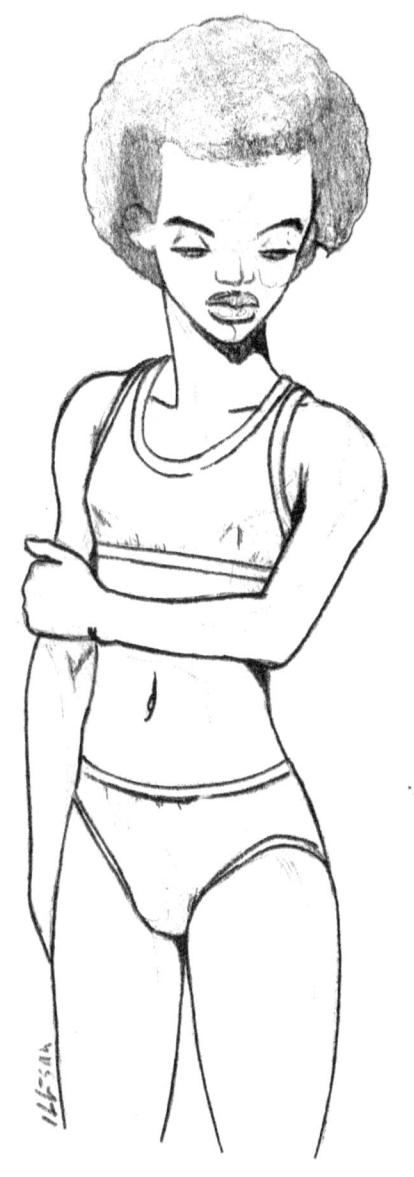

After your breast grows larger you will use a regular bra. A regular bra has two cups, comes in different colors and is fitted by your breast and your chest size. It is very important to get the right size bra because breast grow to different sizes as you get older.

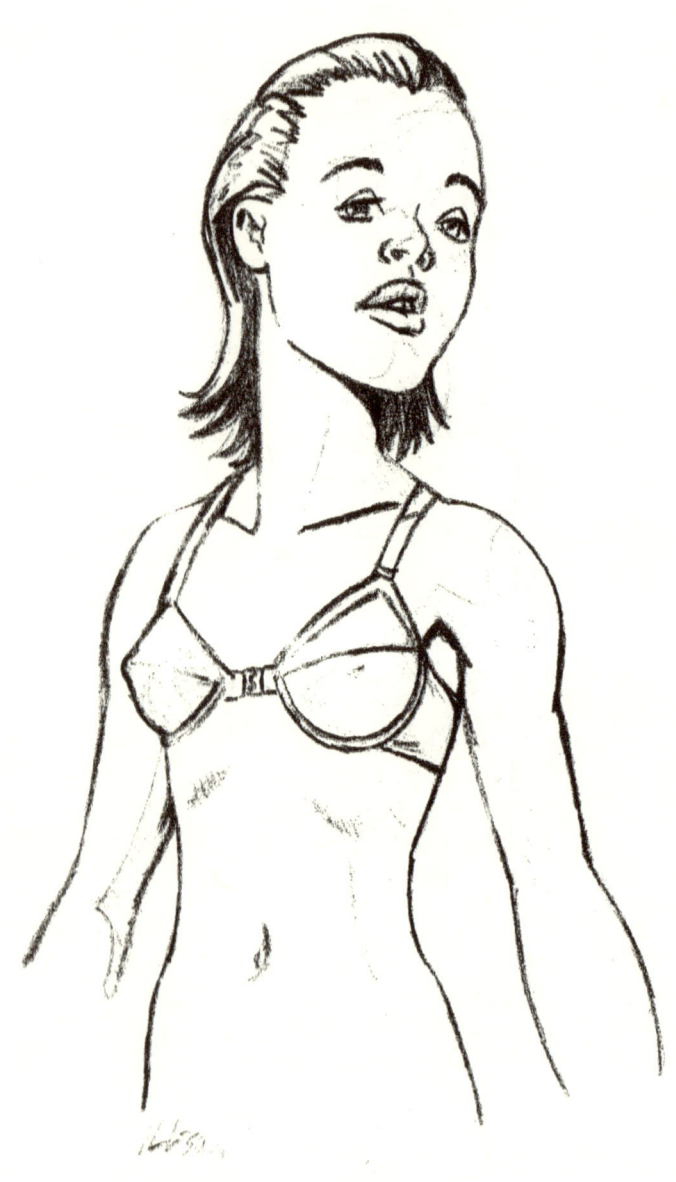

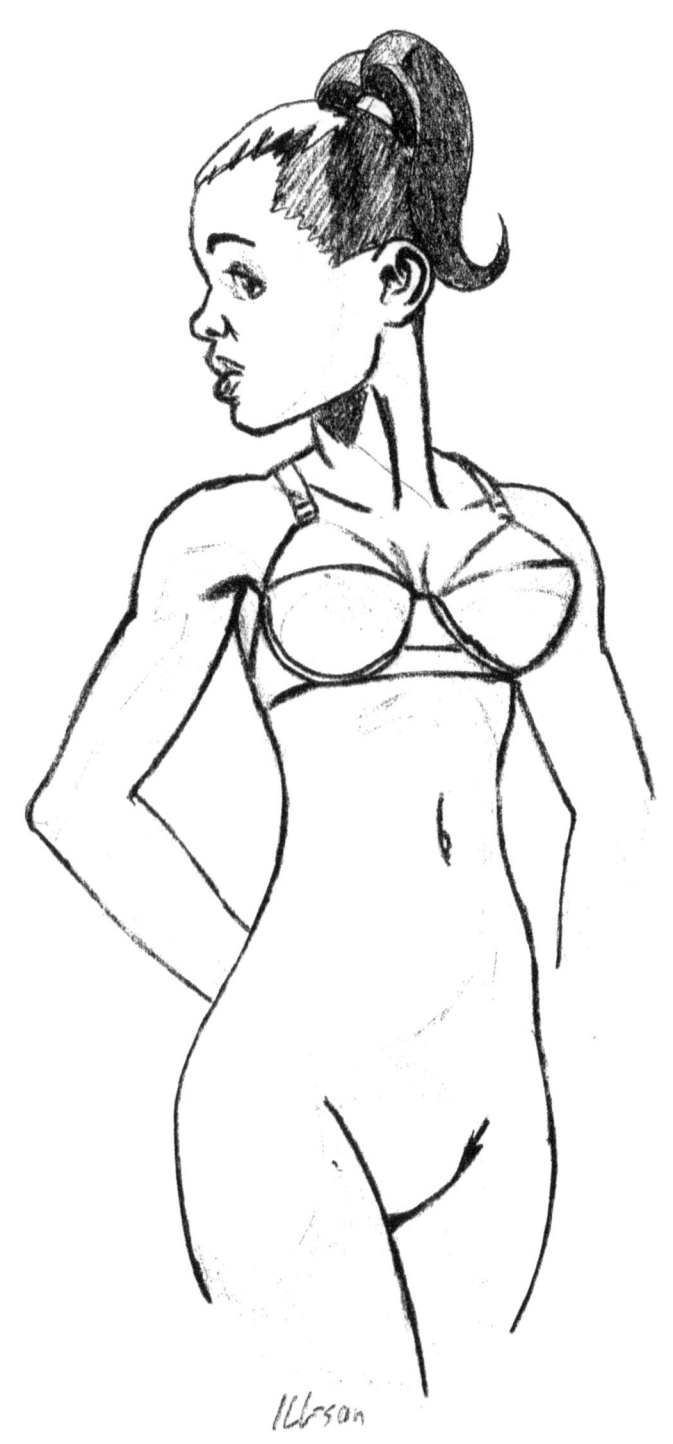

Illusan

There is no such thing as a perfect breast size. All breasts are able; to perform the job God created them for (milk for a baby).

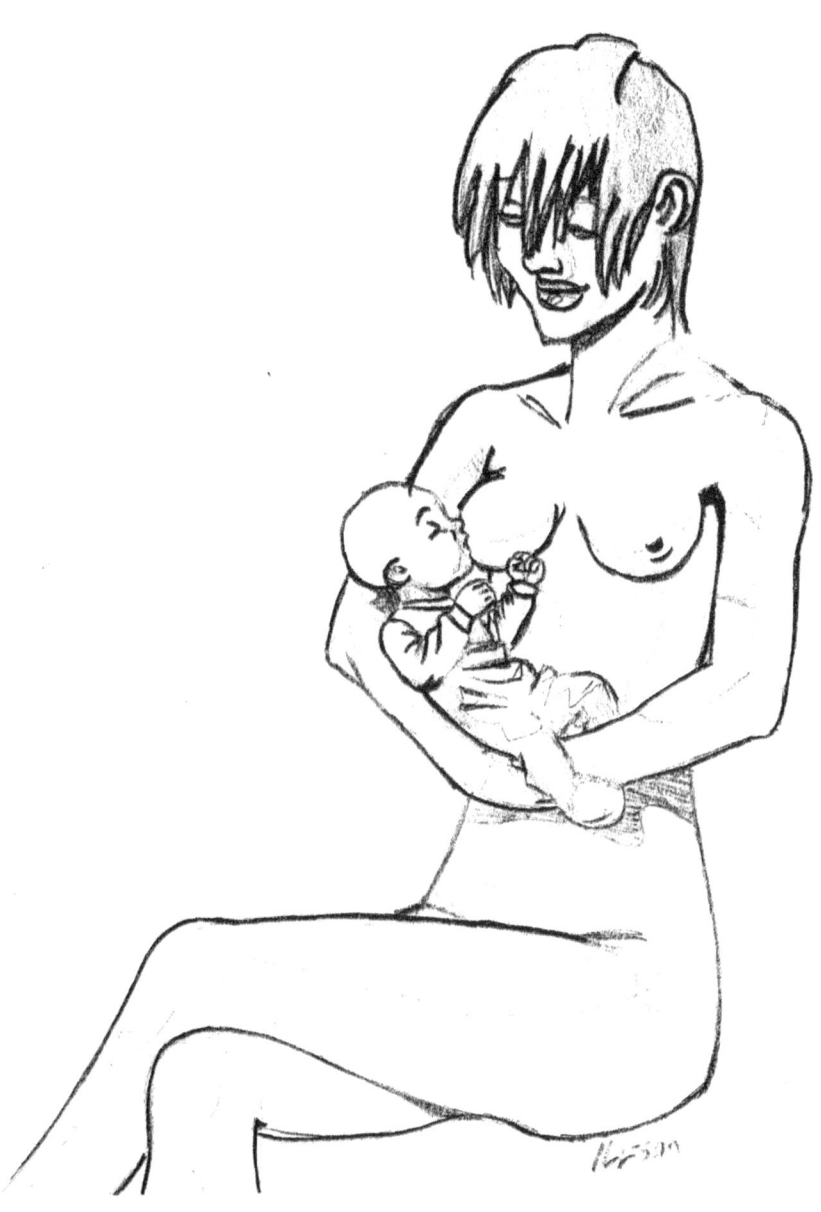

Between the ages of 8 to 12 years old; you will began to feel something leaking from inside your vagina, this is a natural sign of puberty(body change) for a woman. This is called, a discharge; it is a clear or cloudy (white) fluid that is sticky but doesn't smell. A day or so later the discharge will become heavier (leak faster) and turn red, this is blood.

Don't panic this is called, menstruation (period); it is a bright red or dark red flow of blood from inside the vagina for 4-7 days once every month.

You may experience stomach cramps (pain), sadness, anger, bloating (swelling of the stomach), vomiting (throwing up) tenderness in your breast (painful to touch or feeling of tightness). Every woman's experience is different. There are medicines made; to help with all of these symptoms. Your mom will guide you In deciding which ones to try or teach you natural methods, for dealing with the symptoms.

If you are at school when it starts ask for permission to go to the restroom; use toilet tissue as an emergency pad, to prevent the blood from staining your clothes.

Wrap tissue around your wrist and hand until it is thick. It should cover your wrist and hand. Make sure that you wrap the tissue very loose, so that it can be pull off your hand with ease. Place the emergency pad in the center of your panties and pull your panties up; ask for permission to go to the clinic, the nurse might have pads in the clinic for you to use.

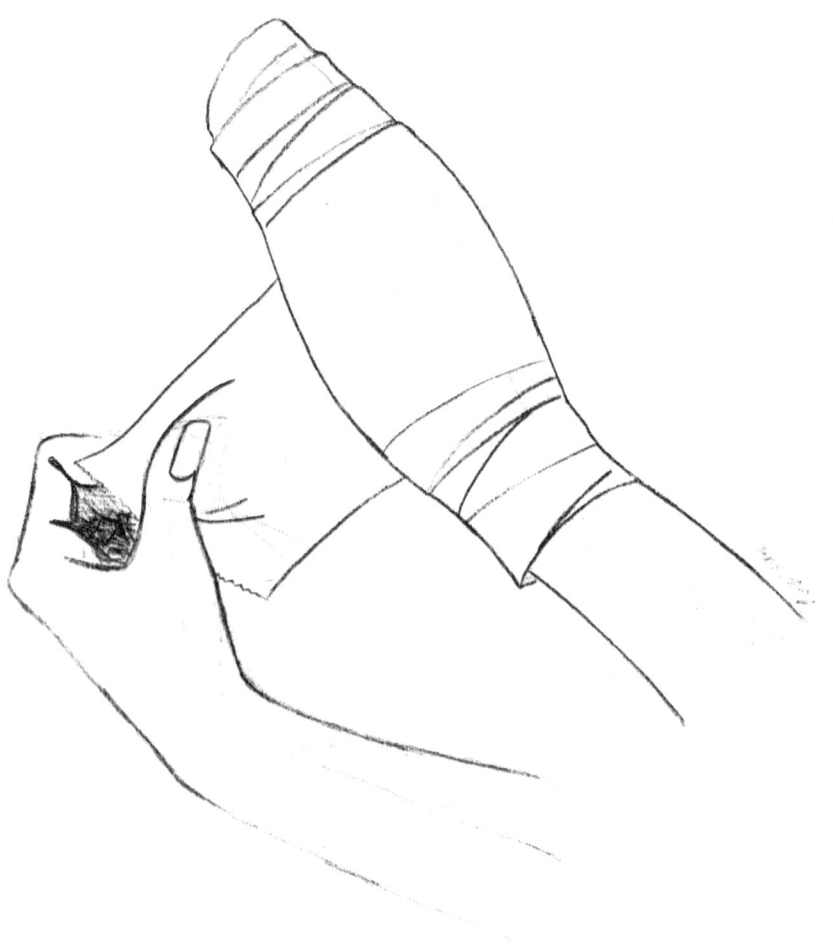

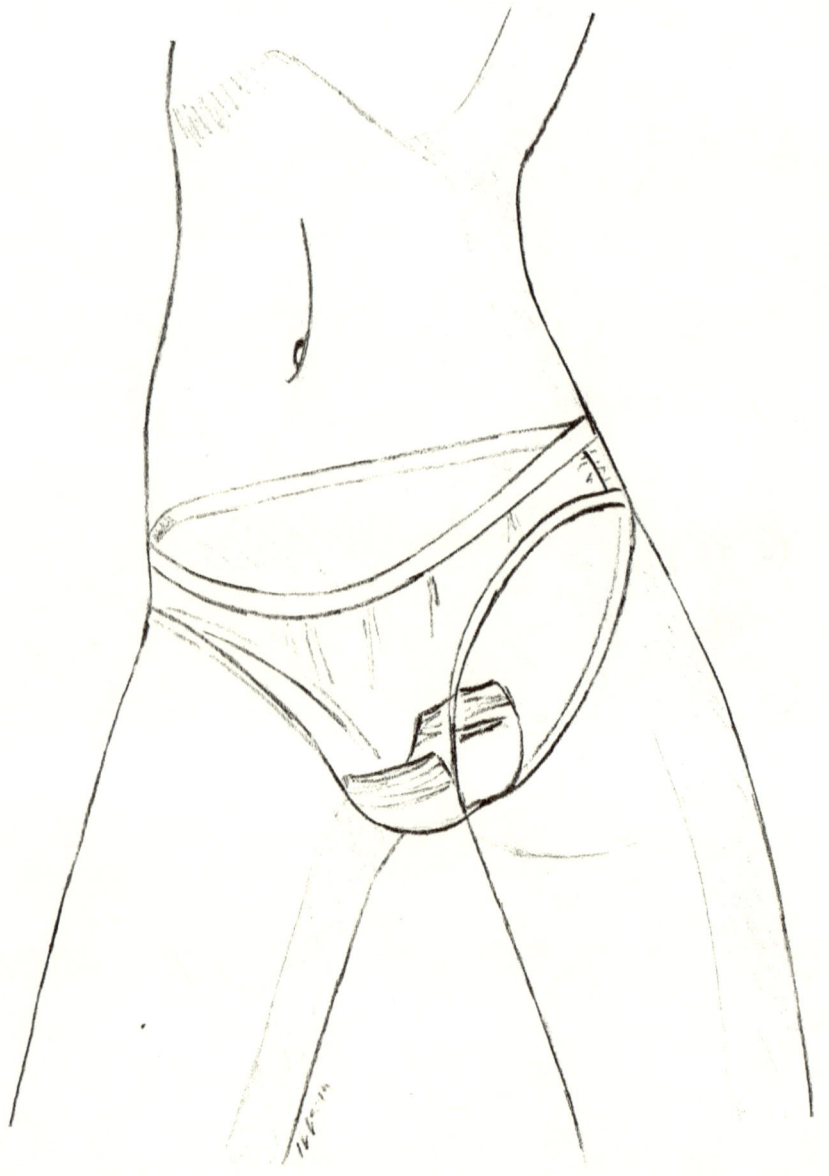

If you have already stained your clothes it is alright, the nurse will call your mom or an adult family member to pick you up. Your mom will teach you how to clean your vagina and help you decide what to use during your menstruation (period).

The process of puberty is complete when you start having periods. If you began to get curious(lots of questions) about sex or think that you feel the need to experiment (try it) with sex, please stop and think, talk to an adult you can trust. They will not get angry with you; they will guide and inform you of some very important information.

If you feel that you can't talk to your family about it, go to the health center in your area; they have information available to teach you. There are two major concerns (things to understand clearly).

You could become pregnant, or pick up a sexually transmitted (from having sex) disease. Don't be afraid, be careful and think before you act.

There are two types of sanitary products a young woman can use during her menstruation (period).

Sanitary Pads: a pad that is placed in the crotch of the panties (between the legs), it has an adhesive strip on the back of it that holds the pad in place, after you press it onto the panties. It absorbs (hold) the blood as it runs down onto the pad. The pad has to be changed at least three or more times a day or it will get too wet and stain your clothes.

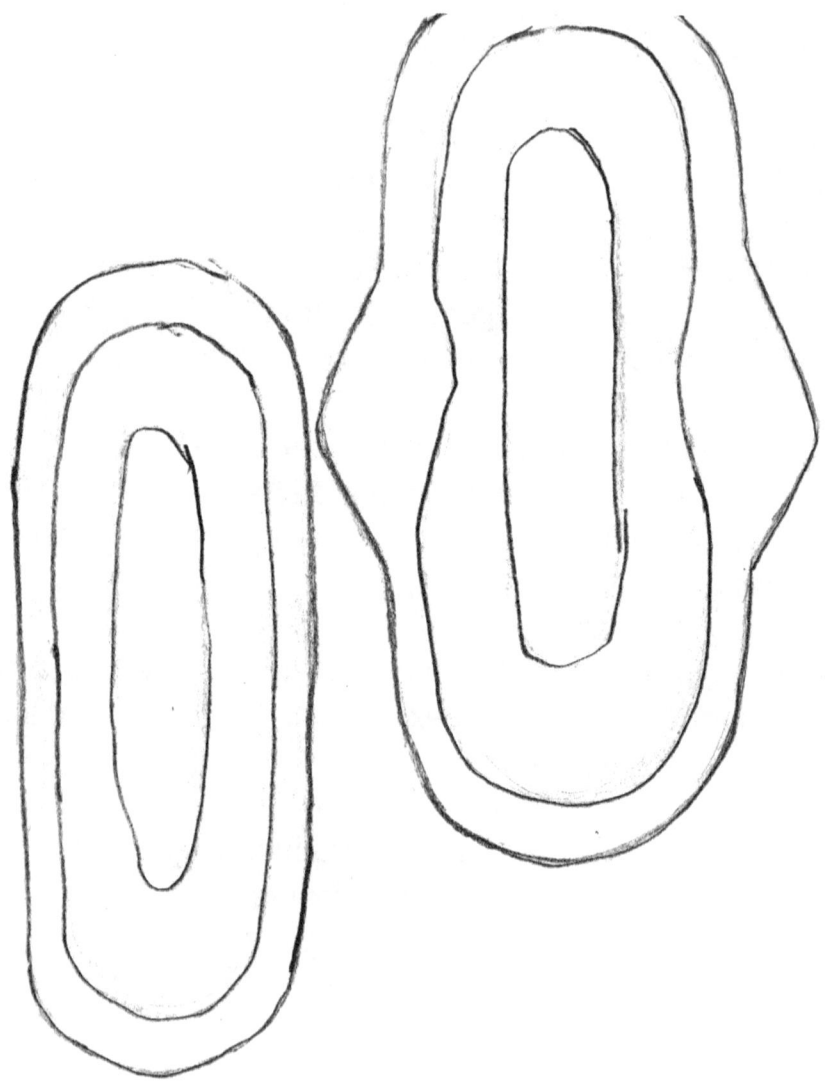

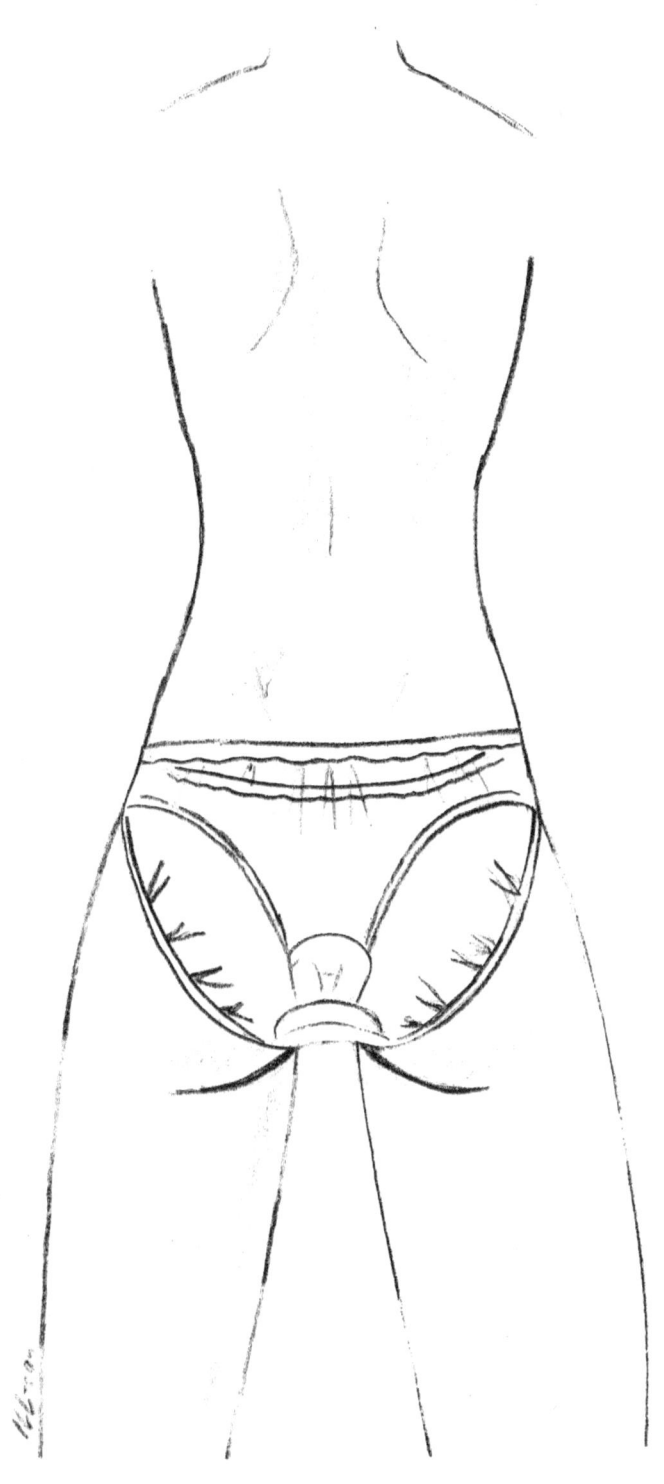

Tampons: a thick circular (round) tube of cotton-like material with a string attached that is inserted (placed) into the vagina with a special tube made of paper or plastic. It absorbs (hold) the blood as it flows down the walls of the vagina and prevents blood from going to the panties. The tampon also has to be changed three or more times a day to prevent staining the panties. The string is attached to aid (help) in removal (pulling out) of the tampon.

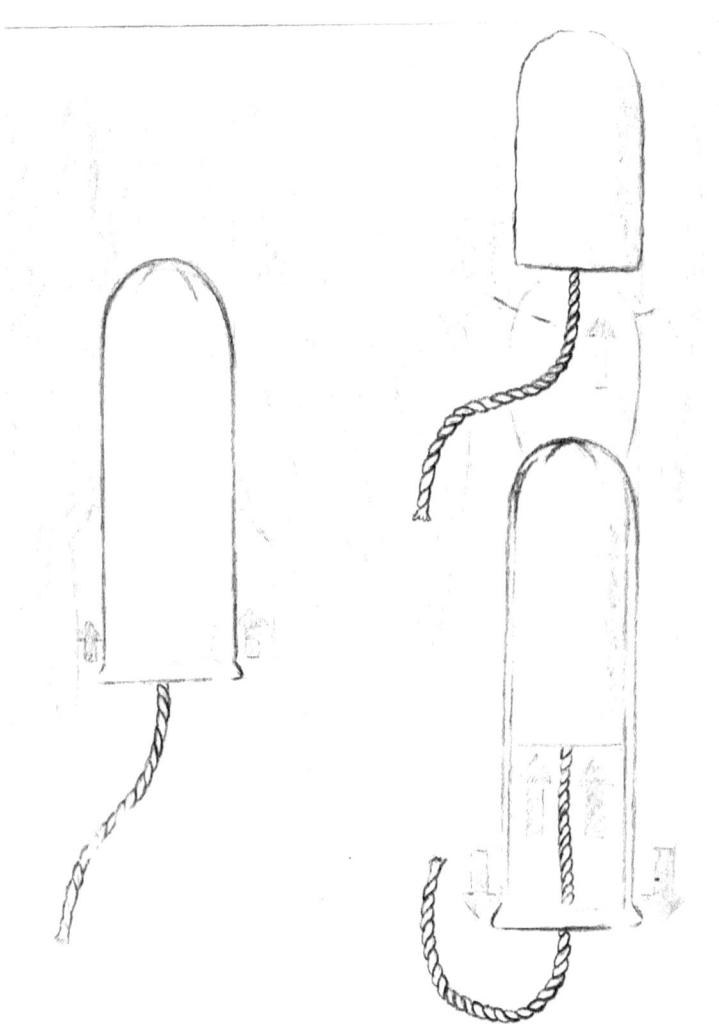

STEP SIX
Body Safety

Only a doctor examining you (checking for injuries), should touch your private body parts; breast, vagina or buttocks (behind). Your body is very special and no one should touch your private body parts.

If this happens Scream, fight, kick and bite them, if you have to, get away from them. If you are Inside a house and you know, that there are other people, in the house also; break things, make as much noise as you can, so someone who's close by will hear you.

Don't be afraid to tell what the person did; even if they said, they will kill your family. They are trying to scare you, so no one will know. If you be brave enough to tell, you'll see that; they are the one who's afraid.

If a stranger grabs you; fight, bite, scratch and kick until you can get away from them. Run and tell an adult what happened. If no adults are around run to a safe place and hide until you see someone that can help. Ask them to call the police for you or go to a pay phone and dial 911, tell the person on the phone what happened, they will talk to you until the police arrive.

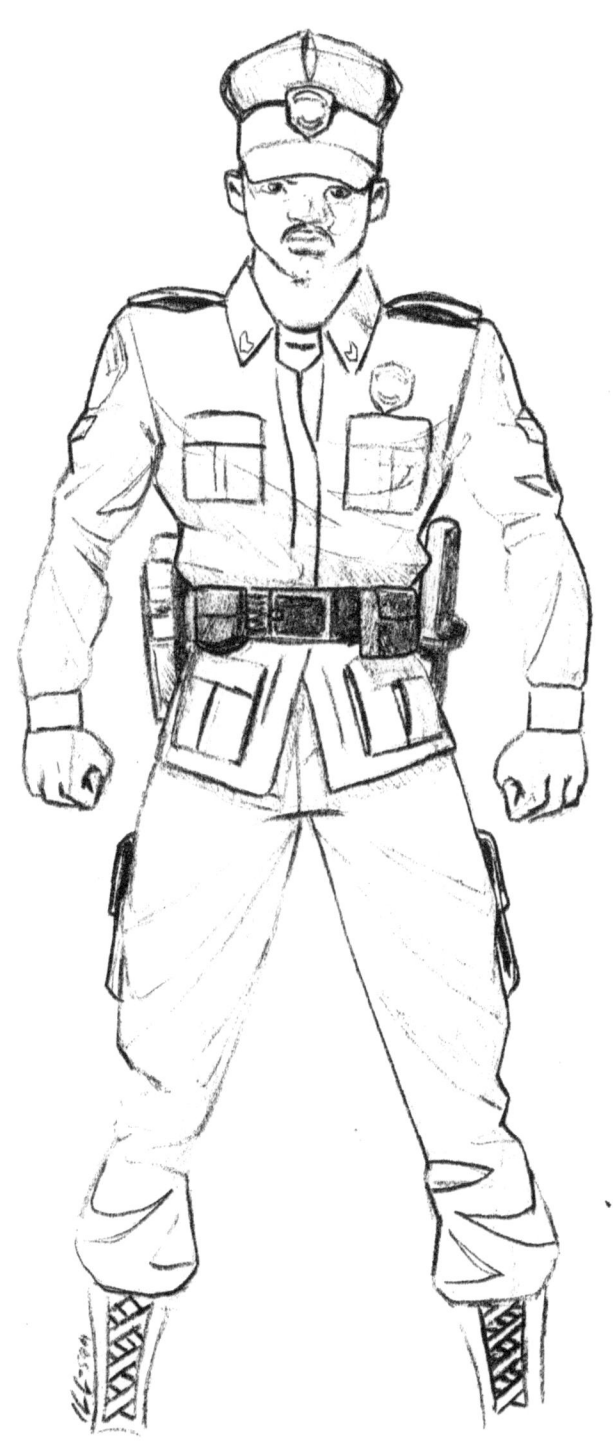

If there is no place to hide, no pay phone and no store close by run to someone's front door and beat on it very hard; Screaming "Help Me!!"as loud as you can until someone comes to help.

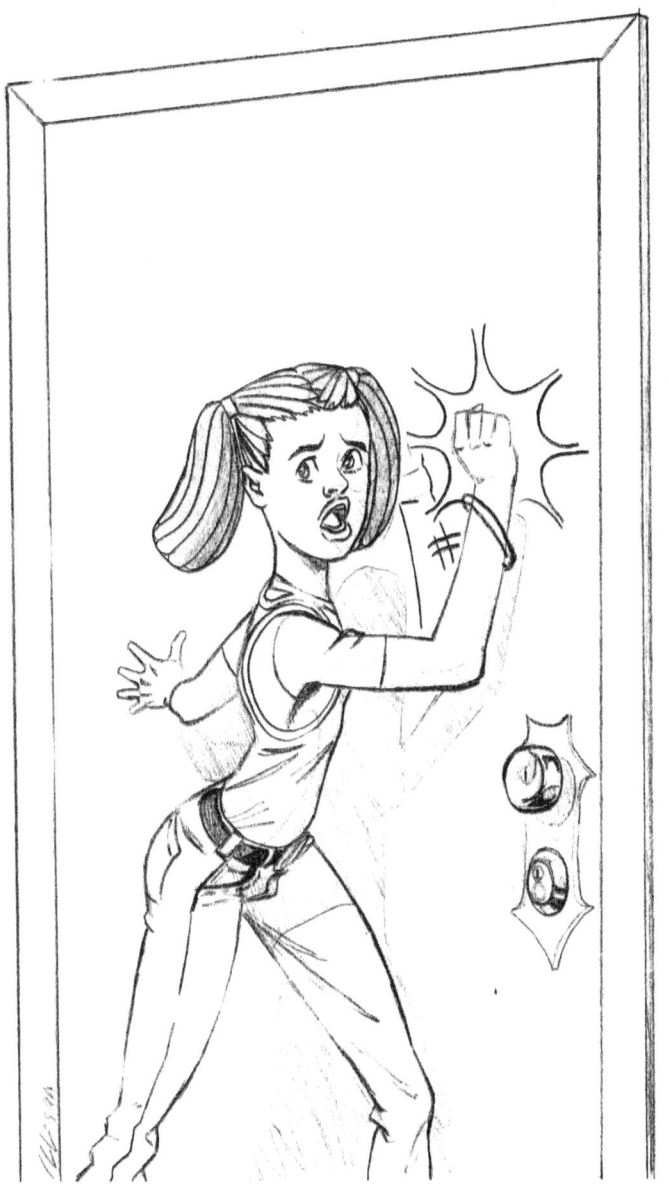

No one should place their mouth on your private body parts, kiss you on your mouth, or ask you to place your mouth on their private body parts. This is very dangerous and you should get away from them fast. Tell somebody what happened right away.

No one should ask you, to pull down your clothes No one should place anything; inside your vagina or buttocks (behind). No one should place a private body part in your mouth no one should allow you to watch any of these things happening.

There are many child predators (people who like to abuse (hurt) children). And sometimes they are not strangers; they may be a friend, a family member, a stranger, a coach, a friend of your parents or a teacher.

If someone seems to be too nice and start to show you things that you know are wrong or you feel uncomfortable about being alone with them. be careful. Tell someone about it right away, they will protect you and keep you safe from danger. If you don't tell anyone nobody will know that you need help.

Not everyone; is a child predator, but pay close attention to the way they act, there are warning signs. If you don't feel safe with a person, stay as far away from them as possible and never allow them to be alone with you. Talk to your mom about this feeling she needs to know in order to protect you.

Keep a positive (good) attitude, care about what you do and how you do it. Something as simple as; how you pick up a piece of paper, represents you (acts or speak for).

Remember; people will only respect you, if you respect yourself. Study hard in school and learn all you can. Knowledge is the most powerful weapon the world has to offer.

Always think before you act and always think for yourself.

Choose a career that fits your likes; if you choose a career because of the money you can make, you may become bored and then poor performance (bad or sloppy work) could cause you to lose your job. When you enjoy what you do; your work stands out, because of the pride you put into doing it.

Be independent (able to take care of yourself) and never completely depend on a man to take care of you. The only power a person has over you is the power that you give them. Don't do anything that doesn't feel right, back away and think about it. Ask yourself questions; talk with an adult about it. No one can live your life for you, and you should not live your life for anyone but yourself.

I'm very sorry; but there is no such thing, as a prince charming that rides a white horse and comes to rescue you. Even if you're lucky enough to find a charming prince; he may one day decide to go his own way. If the love is true; there is no need to try to hang on to someone or thing, they will choose to stay.

There are people; who you will fall in love with, as you grow older, but most of them are placed there, to be a friend and nothing more than that. Acting on emotions (feelings) without thought; often leads us into relationships that are destined (going to) to fail (not work).

GOOD LUCK!!!

Words to Know and Understand

PUBERTY- changes that the body goes through as a person grows from childhood into maturity and becomes able to have children.

VAGINA- a female private body part

FEMALE- a girl or woman

MENSTRUATION- the flow of blood, down through the vagina, that happens every month for 4-7 days.

SANITARY PAD- a pad placed in the crotch of the panties during menstruation to absorb blood.

TAMPON- a tube of cotton-like material that is placed inside the vagina during menstruation to absorb blood.

EMERGENCY PAD- a pad of toilet tissue rolled over the hand and wrist to make thick enough to absorb blood until you get home.

About the Author

She's not an expert nor scholar on child behavior. A woman who has walked a path of low self esteem and depression so deep, that it almost made her give up on life. In the moment of her deepest despair Jesus spoke "write it down". she started writing; thinking that Jesus had told her to write a book. She decided to write about the pain, that was smothering her life. Every available moment was spent writing. Each evening she would review her writing always starting from the beginning.

Eighteen months later it was finished; she mailed out copies to six publishing houses, one was interested but, wanted it rewritten in the third person. She started reviewing it for a rewrite suddenly she realized; she could laugh at the things that once caused her pain. Immediately she knew that God had used her writing to mend her spirit. She stopped all publishing plans and started writing again. Wondering if she could stop or change the pattern of low self esteem among women, How?, When?. Twenty one years have passed and it is finished.

www.ingramcontent.com/pod-product-compliance
Lightning Source LLC
Chambersburg PA
CBHW031242280526
45784CB00004B/1684